INFANT GENDER SELECTION
& PERSONALIZED MEDICINE

INFANT GENDER SELECTION & PERSONALIZED MEDICINE

CONSUMER'S GUIDE

Anne Hart

ASJA Press
New York Lincoln Shanghai

INFANT GENDER SELECTION & PERSONALIZED MEDICINE CONSUMER'S GUIDE

ASJA Press
an imprint of iUniverse, Inc.

iUniverse books may be ordered through booksellers or by contacting:

iUniverse
2021 Pine Lake Road, Suite 100
Lincoln, NE 68512
www.iuniverse.com
1-800-Authors (1-800-288-4677)

ISBN-13: 978-0-595-36539-5
ISBN-10: 0-595-36539-6

Printed in the United States of America

Table of Contents

Chapter One

GENDER SELECTION

ANDREW Y. SILVERMAN, MD, PhD

2 Overhill Road Suite 405

Scarsdale, N.Y. 10583

914–722–9300
http://www.gender-select.com

INTRODUCTION

The desire to influence the sex of the next child is probably as old as recorded history. In the pre-industrialized age, having another son meant that a family had an additional hand to help with manual labor. If an individual could plant and harvest more food than it consumed for survival, a family unit would amass a surplus of food that would help it to survive during the non-growing season, or during times of famine.

In times of war, males were also needed as soldiers to protect their families and their homes. In addition, if you were of royal lineage you needed a son to carry on the family name to subsequent generations. For these reasons, male children were the more desired sex throughout history.

In more modern times, in societies without any form of social security, males were needed for a very different reason. Once a young girl married, she joined the family of her husband, and her labor as well as any income that she earned became part of his family unit. Her aging parents were left to fend for themselves without the benefit of financial security during their old age. On the other hand, sons remained part of an extended family unit, and provided for their aging parents. Today, this is still the case in some societies.

More and more frequently, couples are seeking to select the sex of their next baby. They do so mainly for several reasons. Firstly, couples that have children of the same sex usually want to experience the joy of raising a child of the opposite sex. Secondly, couples that carry a sex-linked disease in their genetic history want to shield their future children from having this disorder.

Lastly, in my experience, women wish to have a daughter of their own, to develop a special mother to daughter relationship. This desire is expressed whether the woman had a good or a bad relationship with her own mother.

HOW IS THE GENDER OF A BABY DETERMINED?

Gender selection is possible because of the way in which sex is determined by our chromosomes. Our bodies are made up of billions of cells. All cells contain 46 rod-like forms arranged in pairs called chromosomes, except for the special reproductive cells (the sperm and egg cells) called gametes, each of which only possess 23 chromosomes.

During fertilization, the gametes combine and restore the normal chromosome number (46) in the embryo. One of these pairs of chromosomes defines the sex of the developing baby. This pair is called the sex chromosome. Each pair of sex chromosomes is made up of an "X and Y" chromosome, which define a male, or an "X and X" chromosome, which define a female. Eggs can only contain X chromosomes, but sperm contain either an X or a Y chromosome.

SEX-LINKED GENETIC DISEASES

Sex-linked genetic diseases include various muscular dystrophies such as Duchenne muscular dystrophy, hemophilia, Charcot-Marie-Tooth disease and color blindness. They are called sex-linked diseases because there is an abnormal gene that is carried on the X chromosome.

A female is made up of two X chromosomes (one from her father and one from her mother). If she inherits one defective X chromosome, she will still be normal as long the second X chromosome is normal. Therefore it is very rare for a female to have a sex-linked disease because the normal X chromosome balances out the abnormal X chromosome. If she has one defective X-chromosome, instead of having the disease, she will be a carrier of this disease and possibly transmit it to her sons.

A male is made up of an X chromosome from his mother, and a Y chromosome from his father. If he inherits a defective X chromosome, he will have the disease because his normal Y chromosome cannot balance his abnormal X chromosome. Diseases linked to the Y chromosome are extremely rare. The best way to prevent transmission of a sex-linked disease is to undergo *in vitro fertilization* with **preimplantation genetic diagnosis (IVF/PGD)**. This process allows the embryologist to screen the embryo for defects before it is transferred to the mother, and a pregnancy occurs.

AUTOSOMAL LINKED GENETIC DISEASES

In each normal human cell there are 23 pairs of chromosomes; one pair is the sex chromosome, and the remainders are called the autosomal chromosomes. These define a person's individual human traits. An autosomal linked genetic disease consists of either additions or deletions of any pair of autosomal chromosomes.

Using fluorescent in situ hybridization (FISH) the embryologist is able to count the number of chromosomes commonly involved in abnormal syndromes such as Chromosome 21 or Chromosome 18. If an embryo shows any of these defects, it is not used for transfer to the uterus.

SINGLE GENE DEFECTS

Some disorders result when a mutation causes a single gene to be damaged or missing. Examples of this kind of disorder are Sickle-Cell Anemia, Tay-Sachs Disease, Thallasemia, Cystic Fibrosis and Down's Syndrome.

To diagnose some of these conditions, the DNA of the embryo is analyzed by chemically producing numerous copies of the suspected gene using the polymerase chain reaction. Embryos that do not have the defect are used for uterine transfer. Not all genetic diseases can be screened, but the list is rapidly expanding.

PROVEN TECHNIQUES OF GENDER SELECTION THE ERICSSON METHOD

Scientists have known for many years that sperm carrying an X chromosome produce females and sperm carrying a Y chromosome produce males. In the early 70's, scientists discovered that sperm samples with high concentrations of either X or Y bearing sperm could be obtained.

In 1975, Ronald J. Ericsson, PhD began clinical studies to determine whether enriched sperm samples would result in offspring of a desired gender. The results were very encouraging and today this procedure is widely accepted by the scientific community. Currently, the Ericsson Method is used in approximately 50 centers in the United States and in many centers worldwide.

How does it work?

Dr. Ericsson devised patented methods by which X and Y sperm can be separated through filtering processes. Sperm are "layered" over a column of human serum albumin and they swim down the gradient where they are collected in the bottom layer.

The fraction of sperm that contains the male (Y) bearing sperm is used for insemination if a boy is desired. It is effective 70–75% of the time. The fraction of sperm that contains the female (X) bearing sperm is used for insemination if a girl is desired. It is effective 70–72% of the time.

Overall, approximately 70–75% of the couples participating in gender selection have a baby of their chosen gender. Over five thousand babies have been born using this method.

Publication:

In 2002, Dr. Silverman and Dr. Ericsson published a study in the journal, *Human Reproduction*, entitled **"Female Sex Selection Using Clomiphene Citrate and Albumin Separation of Sperm"**, which examined the effect of combining the Ericsson Method with Clomid. They demonstrated a 40% increase in the probability of having a girl when Clomid is given to patients selecting for a girl combined with sperm separation.

IVF/PGD GENDER SELECTION TECHNIQUE

After ovarian stimulation, eggs are removed from the mother. These eggs are fertilized in the laboratory with the father's Ericsson Method selected sperm via *in vitro fertilization* (*IVF*) technology. After cell division, the embryos are checked for their sex using preimplantation genetic diagnosis (PGD). Only the embryos of the chosen gender are transferred back to the mother. The number transferred depends upon both medical and social factors. The decision of how many to transfer is individualized for each couple.

IN VITRO FERTILIZATION (IVF)

The term *in vitro* fertilization (*IVF*) literally means "fertilization outside of the body". *IVF* is now routinely used to treat infertility caused by moderate to severe low sperm count, tubal disease and unexplained infertility.

In the *IVF* process, the female receives the follicle stimulating hormone (FSH) by injection. FSH stimulates the recruitment and development of multiple eggs within the ovary. Egg maturity is monitored by the rise in serum estrogen levels, and by measuring follicular growth. FSH is administered until the eggs are mature, and then human chorionic gonadotropin (hCG) is administered 36 hours prior to egg retrieval.

The eggs are retrieved transvaginally (through the vagina) using a needle guided by ultrasound. The male provides a semen sample. This specimen is specially washed and prepared to inseminate the egg. The sperm is then layered on the eggs, and one sperm attaches to and penetrates the egg's membrane (zona pellucida) resulting in fertilization. The fertilized eggs develop into embryos.

The embryos are placed in an incubator and allowed to divide from 3 to 5 days. Where possible, 5-day-old embryos (blastocysts), are transferred to the mother's uterus. Attachment to the uterus results in a developing pregnancy.

When performing *IVF* for gender selection, the embryos are screened for their sex using **preimplantation genetic diagnosis** (PGD). Only embryos of the desired sex will be transferred to the mother's uterus.

PREIMPLANTATION GENETIC DIAGNOSIS (PGD)

PGD is employed in conjunction with *in vitro fertilization*. Couples want to know the sex of their embryos before they are transferred into the mother's uterus, for various reasons. They may want to be sure that only the embryos of the desired sex are transferred to the mother, or if a couple has a high risk of transmitting a **genetic disease,** they may want to make sure they are excluding embryos that have abnormal chromosomes.

PGD enables the embryologist to biopsy the embryo and determine if a disease is present prior to selecting the embryo for transfer to the mother. Every cell in the embryo contains a copy of the genetic makeup of the entire person. PGD begins with an embryo biopsy.

A small hole is made in the egg membrane (zona pellucida) when the embryo has grown to 6–8 cells. One cell is removed from the embryo so that the chromosomes can be examined. Removal of one of these cells does not harm the developing embryo.

In order to check the sex of the embryo, and to exclude embryos that possess sex linked diseases, the cell is analyzed using "fluorescent in situ hybridization" (FISH). FISH is a sophisticated genetic technique used to identify cells possessing chromosomal abnormalities. FISH is also used to identify the male and female embryos allowing the transfer only embryos of the desired sex. Identifying abnormal embryos can prevent the transfer of embryos with sex-linked diseases.

Since only embryos of the desired gender are transferred to the mother's uterus, PGD is extremely effective in determining the unborn offspring's sex.

WHICH GENDER SELECTION OPTION IS RIGHT FOR YOUR FAMILY?

The first step in your search for help with gender selection is to decide how important your next baby's sex is to you and your family. The **Ericsson Method of Gender Selection** increases your odds of having a child of your chosen gender. If you feel that you could not accept a child that may not be the sex that you wanted, then this technique is not for you.

Instead, you should consider the *in vitro fertilization* (*IVF*/PGD) **gender selection** technique since gender selection success rates using this technique approach a 100%. If you are at risk for a sex linked genetic disease, the *IVF*/PGD technique is more effective in preventing the transmission of this disease to your next child.

Gender Selection Success Rates

When couples ask us about success rates, they usually want to know what their chances are of delivering a healthy baby of the desired sex. Success rates depend upon many factors including which procedure is chosen, the couple's age, underlying medical conditions, etc.

Couples who are "reproductively healthy" have a greater chance of conceiving than those with underlying diseases, such as male factor infertility. Couples choosing the **Ericsson Method** of gender selection will undergo an intrauterine insemination cycle(s) of selected sperm.

In any given IUI cycle using unselected sperm when pregnancy occurs, there is a chance that a boy or girl will be conceived. The Ericsson method increases the probability that a boy or girl will be conceived based upon which sperm fraction (albumin separated) is chosen. Approximately 70–75% of the time a couple will have a baby of the selected gender. The percentage for a female offspring increases when **Clomid** is prescribed during the cycle of sperm separation.

Reproductively healthy couples have a 20–25% chance of conceiving in any given month where regular intercourse occurs. Those undergoing **intrauterine insemination** (IUI) with ovulation inducing medications generally have a 25–30% chance of becoming pregnant in any given cycle. Therefore, some couples will require more than one cycle, but most will become pregnant after three attempts. In general, Ericsson Method couples who undergo three cycles of IUI have a >80% of conceiving and a 70–75% chance of obtaining a child of the desired sex.

Preimplantation genetic diagnosis with *IVF* (*IVF*/PGD) yields a higher success rate of gender selection since only embryos of the chosen gender are transferred to the mother. Patients choosing PGD must undergo an *in vitro fertilization* cycle.

Approximately 38% of infertile couples undergoing *IVF* will conceive. This percentage is highly dependent upon several factors including female age, underlying disease(s), and previous treatments.

Couples undergoing *IVF* for gender selection, who are reproductively healthy, should exceed a 38% pregnancy rate. A major determinant of success is the age of the female patient and her ovarian reserve. All *IVF* patients receive injectable follicle stimulating hormone to cause the recruitment and development of multiple follicles.

PGD is performed on the embryos, and only those embryos of the appropriate sex are transferred to the mother. Sometimes it is also possible to freeze embryos for use in future "non-stimulated" cycles. If a reproductively healthy couple undergoes three cycles of *IVF*, they will conceive >80% of the time, and they will have a child of their chosen gender.

GENDER SELECTION COST

The goal of gender selection is to provide the highest quality treatment to each couple so that they may have a healthy baby of their chosen gender. Each couple must undergo an extensive consultation, which helps decide if they are appropriate candidates for the Ericsson Method or *IVF*/PGD.

The Ericsson Method requires intrauterine insemination (IUI) after sperm separation. This simple technique is offered at a reasonable price. The Ericsson Method of gender selection has been available for over 20 years, and there are over 5000 babies born throughout the world using this method. The success rate is between 70–75%, and has been constant over the years.

In vitro fertilization combined with preimplantation genetic diagnosis (*IVF*/PGD) entails the use of the latest advances in reproductive technology. While no method in science can be 100% effective this method approaches as close to 100% as possible. Once the sex of the embryos is determined, only embryos of the desired gender are transferred back to the mother. The cost to deliver advanced reproductive technology is considerably higher than The Ericsson Method. For further information on cost considerations, please contact my office, and we will be happy to discuss them with you.

*   *   *

Curriculum Vitae and Publications of Dr. Andrew Y Silverman, MD, PhD.

Andrew Y. Silverman, MD, PhD

DATE AND PLACE OF BIRTH: June 10, 1943—New York City, New York

EDUCATION:
College: Dartmouth College, Hanover, New Hampshire, A.B.   1961–1965
Medical School: S.U.N.Y. at Buffalo, School of Medicine,
Buffalo, New York, M.D.   1965–1972

Graduate School: S.U.N.Y. at Buffalo, School of Medicine,
Department of Microbiology, Buffalo,
New York, Ph.D.   1966–1972

INTERNSHIP: Department of Obstetrics and Gynecology, University
Michigan Medical Center, Ann Arbor, Michigan   1972–1973

RESEARCH ASSOCIATE: National Cancer Institute, National
Institutes of Health, Bethesda, Maryland   1973–1975

RESIDENT: Department of Obstetrics and Gynecology, McGill
University, Montreal, Quebec, Canada   1975–1978

FELLOWSHIP: Reproductive Endocrinology, Department of
Obstetrics and Gynecology, The University of Texas Health
Science Center at San Antonio, Texas   1978–1981

CERTIFICATION: Diplomat, National Board of Medical Examiners   1973
Diplomat, Licensure Medical Council Canada   1976
Diplomat, American Board of Obstetrics and
Gynecology   1983
The Society of Reproductive Surgeons   1993

LICENSED: Maryland, 1974; Quebec, Canada, 1976; Texas 1978;
New York, 1984

HONORS:
Third Prize, Current Clinical and Basic Investigation, presented at the 27th Annual Meeting of The American College of Obstetrics and Gynecology, 1979 Selected as a participant of the Mead Johnson Perinatal and Development Medicine Symposium, Marco Island, Florida, December 2–6, 1979

APPOINTMENTS:
Assistant Professor of Obstetrics and Gynecology, The University
of Texas Health Science Center at San Antonio, Texas   1978–1984
Chief of Gynecology, Audie Murphy Veterans Administration Hospital,
San Antonio, Texas   1979–1983
Director of Human In Vitro Fertilization, Department of Obstetrics and
Gynecology, The University of Texas Health Science Center at San
Antonio, Texas   1981–1983
Clinical Assistant Professor of Obstetrics and Gynecology, New York
Medical College, Valhalla, New York   1985–
Medical Committee of Planned Parenthood of Westchester   1987–
Director of the Medical Committee of Planned Parenthood of
Hudson Peconic, Inc.   1994–2000

ORGANIZATIONS:
American College of Obstetricians and Gynecologists
    Junior Fellow   1973–1983
    Fellow   1984–
The American Society of Reproductive Medicine   1984–
American Association for the Advancement of Science   1981–1985
San Antonio Obstetrical and Gynecological Society   1982–1984
Bexar County Medical Society   1983–1984
The Endocrine Society   1983–1990
Westchester County Medical Society   1985–1987
New York County Medical Society   1987–1989
The Society of Reproductive Surgeons   1993–

AD HOC EDITOR:
Fertility and Sterility   1989–
International Journal of Gynecology   1981–

HOSPITAL AFFILIATIONS:
Westchester (County) Medical Center, Valhalla, New York   1985–
White Plains Hospital Center, White Plains, New York   1989–

*   *   *

Andrew Y. Silverman, MD, PhD

PUBLICATIONS

Papers:

1. Silverman, A.Y. and Boylan, J.W.: Further studies on renal glucose transport in Squalus acanthias: Effect of epinephrine. Bulletin of Mt. Desert Island Biological Laboratory, p. 36, 1966.

2. Silverman, A.Y., Yagi, Y., Pressman, D., Ellison, R.R., and Tormey, D.C.: Monoclonal IgA & IgM in the serum of a single patient. (SC). III. Immuno-fluorescent identification of cells producing IgA & IgM. J. Immunology 110: 350, 1973.

3. Watanabe, S., Silverman, A.Y., Yagi, Y. and Yamamura, Y.: Studies On membrane bound immunoglobulin of human lymphoid cell line. I. Proceeding of the IIIrd Annual Meeting of the Japanese Society of Immunology, p. 351, 1973.

4. Silverman, A.Y.: Aspects of Immunoglobulin synthesis in human lymphoid cells established in culture. Ph.D. thesis, copyright 1975.

5. Howk, R.S., Anisowica, A., Silverman, A.Y., Parks, W.P. and Scolnick E.M.: Distribution of murine type B and type C viral nucleic acid sequences in template active and inactive chromatin. Cell 4:321, 1975.

6. Silverman, A.Y., Artinian, B. and Sabin, M.: A case report of a serous cystadenofibroma of the fallopian tube. Am. J. Obstet. Gynecol. 130:593, 1978.

7. Murphy, B.E.P. and Silverman, A.Y.: A comparison of glucocorticoid conjugates with other indices of fetal maturation. Obstet. Gynecol. 54: 35, 1978.

8. Steger, R.W., Silverman, A.Y., Siler-Khodr, T.M. and Asch, R.H.: The effect of delta0-tetrahydrocannabinol on the positive and negative feedback control of luteinizing hormone release. Life Sciences 27: 1911, 1980.

9. Silverman, A.Y., Smith, C.G., Siler-Khodr, T.M. and Asch, R.H.: hCG Blocks the estrogen-induced LH release in long-term castrated Rhesus Monkeys: Evidence for an ultrashort-loop negative feedback. Fertil. Steril. 35:74, 1981.

10. Steger, R.W., Silverman, A.Y., Johns, A. and Asch, R.H.: Interaction Of cocaine and delta9-tetrahydrocannabinol (THC) with the hypothalamic-hypophysial axis of the female rat. Fertil. Steril. 35: 567, 1981.

11. Steger, R.W., Silverman, A.Y., and Asch, R.H.: Glucocorticoid suppression of pituitary prolactin release in the non-human primate. J. Clin. Endocrinol. Metab. 53:1167, 1981.

12. Silverman, A.Y., Darnell, B.J., Montiel, M.M., Smith, C.G. and Asch, R.H.: Response of rhesus monkey lymphocytes to short-term administration of THC. Life Sci. 30:107–109, 1982.

13. Silverman, A.Y.: The success rate of in vitro fertilization: What can the patient expect? Am. J. Obstet. Gynecol. 144:360–361, 1982.

14. Silverman, A.Y. Schwartz, S.L. and Steger, R.W.: A quantitative Difference between immunologically and biologically active prolactin in Hypothyroid patients. J. Clin. Endocrinol. Metab. 55:272–275, 1982.

15. Herbert, D.C. and Silverman, A.Y.: Topographical distribution of the gonadotrophs, mammotrophs, somatotrophs and thyrothrops in the pituitary gland of the baboon. Cell Tissue Res. 230:233–238, 1983.

16. Cameron, I.L., Lum, J.B., Nations, C., Asch, R.H. and Silverman, A.Y. assay for characterization of human follicular oocyte maturation inhibitor using Xenopus oocytes. Biol. Reprod. 28:817–822, 1983.

17. Steger, R.W., DePaolo, L.V., Asch, R.H. and Silverman, A.Y.: interactions of delta9-tetrahydrocannabinol (THC) with hypothalamic neurotransmitters controlling luteinizing hormone and prolactin release. Neuroendocrinology 37:361–370, 1983.

18. Silverman, A.Y. and Greenberg, E.I.: Absence of a segment of the proximal portion of a fallopian tube. Obstet. Gynecol. 62 (Suppl): 908–918, 1983.

19. Ellsworth, L.R., Balmaceda, J.P., Schenken, R.S., Silverman, A.Y., Prihoda, T.J. and Asch, R.H.: Human chorionic gonadotropin and steroid concentrations in human follicular fluid in relation to follicular Size and oocyte maturity in stimulated ovarian cycles. Acta Europa Fertilitatis. 15, #5, 1984.

20. Silverman, A.Y., Renzin, S., Ratz, O., Back, F., Kaali, S.G. and Landesman, R.: Pregnancy obtained by in vitro fertilization in an ambulatory-care surgical facility. New York State J. of Medicine 85:654-655, 1985.

21. Silverman, A.Y., Stephens, S.R., Drouin, M.T., Zack, R.G., Osborne, J. And Ericsson, S.A.: Female sex selection using clomiphene citrate and Albumen separation of human sperm. Human Reproduction 17:no. 5, 1254–1256, 2002.

Chapters:

1. Asch, R.H. and Silverman, A.Y.: Galactorrhea. In: The Gynecologic Patient: A Rational Approach to Diagnosis and Treatment. C.J. Pauerstein (ed.), Gruen & Stratton, Inc., New York. 1982 pp. 201–227.

2. Pauerstein, C.J., Silverman, A.Y. and Eddy, C.A.: Ovum transport and implantation. In: In Vitro Fertilization and Embryo Transfer. Academic Press, Inc., London, 1983, pp. 229–237.

*   *   *

Andrew Y. Silverman, MD., PhD.

Abstracts:

1. Silverman, A.Y. and Murphy, B.E.P.: A comparison of glucocorticoid sulfates (GCS) with other indices of fetal maturation in amniotic fluid from a group of high-risk pregnancies. The 29th Annual Meeting of the American College of Obstetricians and Gynecologists, New York, March 21–April 5, 1979.

2. Silverman, A.Y., Smith, C.G. and Asch, R.H.: Evidence for a LH ultra-short-loop negative feedback (USNF) in castrated rhesus monkeys. The 28th Annual Meeting of the Pacific Coast Fertility Society, Scottsdale, Arizona, October 15–19th, 1979.

3. Silverman, A.Y., Steger, R.W., Schwartz, S.L. and Asch, R.H.: A difference of immunologically and biologically active prolactin in hypothyroid patients. The 29th Annual Meeting of the Pacific Coast Fertility Society, Rancho Mirage, California, October 14–18, 1981.

4. Silverman, A.Y., Asch, R.H., Lum, J.B. and Cameron, I.L.: Presence Of human oocyte maturation inhibitor (OMI) in the follicular fluid from graffian follicles. The 30th Annual Meeting of the Pacific Coast Fertility Society, Scottsdale, Arizona, October 13.17, 1982.

5. Steger, R.W., DePaola, L., Asch, R.H. and Silverman, A.Y.: hypothalamic mediation of the inhibitory affects of delta9-tetrahydrocannabinol (THC)

on steroid-induced gonadotropin surges. The 65th Annual Meeting of The Endocrine Society, San Antonio, Texas, June 8–10, 1983.

6. Silverman, A.Y., Miller, J.P., DeLee, J.C. and Adams, N.D.: Amenorrhea and decreased bone density in an 18 year-old athlete. ACOG District VII Annual Meeting, Houston, Texas, October 2–5, 1983.

7. Ellsworth, L.R., Balmaceda, J.P., Schenken, R.S., Silverman, A.Y. and Asch, R.H.: Human chrionic gonadotropin (hCG) and steroid concentrations in human preovulatory follicular fluid. The 31st Annual Meeting of the Society for Gynecologic Investigation. San Francisco, California, March 21–24, 1984.

Chapter Two

Testing Your Genes for Personalized Medicine

This book is meant to empower the general consumer with knowledge about infant gender selection, personalized medicine, DNA testing for predisposition to diseases, risk, or for deep maternal and paternal ancestry when written records are absent. It's also about matching your foods, medicines, treatments, cosmetics, and lifestyles to your individual genetic signature. And it explores how or whether different drugs and dosages or even foods, affect different races or ethnicities. Where are the newest trends pointing?

At home-genetic testing needs watchdogs, Web sites, and guidebooks to interpret test results in plain language for those with no science background. Online, you'll find genetic tests for ancestry or for familial (genetic, inherited) disease risks.

What helpful suggestions do general consumers with no science background need to consider? What's new in medical marketing is genetic testing online for *predisposition* to diseases—such as breast cancer or blood conditions. Kits usually are sent directly to the consumer who returns a mouthwash or swab DNA sample by mail.

What type of training do healthcare teams need in order to interpret the results of these tests to consumers? Once you receive the results of online genetic testing kits, how do you interpret it? If your personal physician isn't yet trained to interpret the results of online genetic tests, how can you find a healthcare professional that is trained?

If you're more interested in genetic testing for ancestry, do you go to a genealogist or to a geneticist to interpret the results? What if your interest is in genetic testing for disease risks? Do you go to a physician, a nutritionist, a genetics counselor, or a geneticist to find out how certain foods, medicines, dosages, or other products affect your individual genetic expression?

Online firms increasingly market tests that reveal predisposition to diseases. They show risk rather than a sentence that you'll get the disease. Some of these genetic tests offered online show predisposition to breast cancer, blood clotting, or other genetic tendencies. Each day, there's another genetic discovery ranging from varying the dosages of medicines according to one's ethnicity or race mixture to examining the effects of certain foods on certain peoples based on genetic test results. One example would be lactose intolerance—inability to digest milk without symptoms.

Since the human genome code was cracked in the year 2000, scientists have been publishing the results of genetic research, including maps of human, animal, and plant genes. Genetic tests are easy to take. You rub a felt or cotton swab around inside of your mouth and mail it to the testing company according to directions. Your results can be read online. How do you interpret those results?

If you take the results to your doctor, and your physician has never been trained to interpret the results in plain language, you'll need some guidance on how to choose a physician or genetics counselor who has the current training. If the results also were interpreted online, you wouldn't need to visit your physician to get the big picture. So when you take your test, and see your results online, write to your company asking them to also put online samples of how results are interpreted. Your individual genes will be different from someone else's, but at least you will be able to see in plain language how someone else's tests were interpreted. So far, no detailed interpretations of tests for disease of anonymous individuals are specifically put online for the consumer with little or no science background. Will this day be soon arriving?

What's certain is that DNA tests for predisposition to diseases are affordable and not expensive. Your genetic test results that you take from online testing firms are **not** put into your permanent medical records. That way, private information won't get into the hands of anyone who requests your medical records, like insurance companies and employers chomping at the bit to find out to what you're predisposed.

I like the online approach because it validates your family history. Predictive medicine is the cure of the future. There is a high demand for breast cancer genetic tests through online testing kits. Predictive medicine is growing rapidly in revenue and in consumer demand. **If you want to find out what a company's revenues are, begin your research by looking at any company's regulatory filings.** Under the banner "predictive medicine," you can start your search as a consumer. What sells the most? So far, breast cancer genetic tests are popular.

Look for a genetic testing company online that employs its own physicians and genetics counselors who are trained to interpret in plain language to consumers with no science background on how to interpret the results of the specific the types of tests offered. Look for companies that work with doctor's orders and signed informed consent documents for each test.

What you need before you start your research as a consumer of predictive medicine is to be able to reach professionals online. You may even live or work in an area where it's hard to find a doctor. You need to be able to see your results online and be able to reach someone who can interpret those results in plain language so you can follow the diet, dosage, or lifestyle that best suits your individual genetic expression.

It's all about expertise in interpreting the results DNA or other genetic marker tests. Who has the expertise, and how do general consumers find that expert online? With so few genetic counselors available who are trained (approximately 2,000) how will a genetic counselor explain the results of a genetic test to see how your body responds to various medicine dosages when that counselor is trained to talk about pregnancy?

The jobs for many genetics counselors currently are with firms that work with women that have pregnancy concerns. If you want to research this issue on your own, start with the studies of primary care physicians done by the Center for Disease Control and Prevention.

Focus on the particular studies of primary care physicians' inability to handle the overwhelming demand for genetic testing but only after the genetic tests were advertised in the media. Note that these types of studies are usually restricted to certain parts of the country. Any good university library or medical school library has articles and studies on their shelves, but few consumers take the time to research studies concerning the demand for genetic testing, particular tests marketed online. Medical marketing focuses more on TV and magazine advertising of drugs rather than marketing online genetic testing kits in popular magazines.

Is there a way consumers can catch up with technology? Yes, online, if the online material is perceived and verified as credible. So what can the consumer with no science background do—get involved in public policy and team up with scientists? That's the first step—empowering yourself by learning to interpret complex DNA test results if only for your individual markers.

You'll need a physician trained to interpret genetic test results and a genetics counselor on your team, but you need this type of team consisting of consumer and professional—online together. No doctor is going to handle a flood of demand for genetic test kit interpretation. What can you do? You can offer an online company that does nothing but interpret the results and acts as a middle person connecting consumer and physician. What you can do is start that type of online company provided the better mouse trap, that is, the online company that will interpret DNA tests given by other online companies.

Another position the general consumer can take is to seek to regulate the market. You can open a company that validates the online companies. And if you don't want to open a company, you can research and offer information to consumers and to physicians. What if you are a consumer who only wants a genetic test to find out whether you're predisposed to a specific disease such as breast cancer? Here's a company that I highly recommend, DNA Direct, located in San Francisco. What I like about this company is that it is online and has assembled a dedicated staff of genetic and medical experts. DNA Direct provides direct-to-consumer personalized genetic testing services that help consumers put their genes in context with their overall health, lifestyle, and environment.

About DNA Direct

The results of each test are paired with an in-depth Personalized Report that combines an individual's unique test results, lifestyle and health concerns with a practical plan for action. Each report includes scientific research and extensive resources. In addition, customers are encouraged to call or email DNA Direct's genetic experts for further discussion, interpretation and/or resources and information. DNA Direct believes that testing is about empowerment—your body and your health are ultimately your responsibility.

And your genes offer tremendous insight and play a vital role in each personal, medical and lifestyle choice. DNA Direct is a privately held company, incorporated in the fall of 2003, located in San Francisco, California. The company is staffed by a group of dedicated individuals and genetic experts committed to building a genetic testing service that empowers health care consumers.

Genetic testing offers information that can help people make informed decisions about medical management and lifestyle choices. In the current healthcare model, not everyone has access to genetic testing for a variety of reasons.

In genetics publishing, this is the era of making the Web pay. DNA-driven ancestry, molecular anthropology, and genealogy-related books reached the general consumer market in 2002. In book publishing, each year is the year of the special interest book. The mid-nineties, particularly 1996, emphasized Internet-related books. The eighties focused on the recovery book. Angel books flooded the stores in the late nineties. The turn of the millennium saw an increase in popular diary novel and true life story memoirs. Currently, the human genome—DNA is big news and big publishing. Online genetic testing with direct-to-consumer contact provides an open door to predictive medicine research.

As mandated by medical professional societies, genetic tests must often be ordered by a physician and test results are interpreted by a genetic counselor, geneticist, or specialist. In some states, genetic testing must be accompanied by an in-person genetics evaluation and/or genetic counseling appointment.

This approach is limited by the fact that there are only 1,200 medical geneticists and just over 2,000 genetic counselors in the US, most often based in urban areas. The number and type of genetic tests are growing exponentially, and they provide a unique opportunity for consumers to learn more about their health.

DNA Direct's Solution

DNA Direct provides individuals with access to confidential genetic testing using quality-assured tests from CLIA-certified labs. DNA Direct's Web-based genetic testing service redefines traditional, face-to-face genetic counseling and allows individuals to be proactive in managing their care. *Why test?* People seek genetic testing for a variety of reasons, including medical, social, emotional and financial.

✓ Knowledge about your genes can help you make better decisions for your health and for your family.

✓ The results of a test can give you specific information about your unique body—and you could be empowered to take actions that really make changes in your life.

✓ Your genes combine with other factors to influence your health. To understand what your test results really mean, they need to be interpreted in the context of your overall health, lifestyle, and environment.

✓ From peace-of-mind to prevention or treatment, genetic information can tailor your healthcare to best suit your needs.

How Testing Works:

DNA Direct's genetic testing services are high quality, confidential and convenient. The company offers genetic tests that are scientifically proven and performed by CLIA-certified labs. As new tests become commercially available, DNA Direct has the ability to evaluate and make them available to consumers. DNA Direct's solution is simple, easy to use and a certified genetic expert is available to answer questions at any point in the decision, testing, results and reporting process (M-F, 9:00 a.m.—5 p.m. PST). Here's how it works:

Step 1: Get Informed

Learn about genetic testing and determine whether a genetic test is right for you. Knowing whether a medical condition has a genetic basis can be the first step in taking action to live a longer, healthier life. The Web site features:

✓ Information about specific genetic tests
✓ A Resource Center with information on genetic conditions, basic genetic concepts, and family stories
✓ "Why Take a Genetic Test?" and other information on testing

Step 2: Purchase a Test Online, Submit a Sample

The test is easy, painless and completely anonymous with DNA Direct's secure ordering process. Once ordered, a test kit is sent to you. Each kit contains:

✓ A cheek-swab home test kit *
✓ A postage-paid return envelope
✓ An informed consent form

To test, simply swab the inside of your cheeks with the test kit swabs. Then mail them to the lab in the envelope provided. If you have already had genetic testing, DNA Direct's experts can prepare a Personalized Report using existing test results.

Privacy is of the utmost importance. All personal information is and remains private. Within two business days of purchase, you will receive a genetic test kit in a discreet mailer.

Step 3: View Results & Personalized Report

When the lab result is ready (7–10 days after sample is received), you will receive an email with a password-protected link to your Personalized Report. Simply click on the link, and log in using the secure email and password. The report can be printed, referenced later or shared with others, such as a physician.

Genes are only one piece of the health puzzle. A person's history, lifestyle and other factors also play an important role. The Personalized Report is an essential component to putting your genes in context and giving him or her tools and information to make informed choices. All DNA Direct's genetic tests are accompanied

---

* Some tests require a blood sample. For these, DNA Direct provides simple tools to help locate a local clinic affiliate to have a simple, anonymous blood sample taken.

by individually tailored Web reports, which interpret test results in the context of these factors, and explain them in plain English. A Personalized Report includes:

✓ Lab results and an easy-to-understand explanation of the results.

✓ Suggestions on how to improve your health and reduce your risk.

✓ What your results mean to your family, how to talk with your family or doctor

✓ A physician's letter should you wish to consult your doctor

✓ Links to other resources, further reading and support services.

✓ Toll-free access to DNA Direct's genetic experts for additional support and education. DNA Direct's certified genetic counselors are available from 9:00 a.m. to 5:00 p.m. PST, Monday-Friday, 1.877.646.0222 or via email at expert@dnadirect.com.

DNA Direct's Commitment to Your Well Being

Genetics is all DNA Direct does. Its dedication means consumers benefit from the latest research and developments in this fast-moving area of science. DNA Direct collects genetic news and scientific updates of interest to our customers. The DNA Direct Web site offers information on basic genetics, diseases and conditions, FAQs, the latest research, and more.

DNA Direct brings its customers the latest news on their health and genetic concerns, and it encourages them to stay up-to-date on the health news and medical research that's most important to them by subscribing to DNA Direct's News Alerts (no personal information, including email addresses is ever shared). For additional information about DNA Direct, services and support, call 1–877–646–0222.

DNA Direct leverages the Internet to offer personalized genetic tests to help consumers make more informed healthcare choices. DNA Direct's confidential genetic testing offers consumers unparalleled access and insight with personalized reports and genetic expert support.

According to DNA Direct's press release of February 9, 2005, the Internet has clearly become a valued resource for consumers seeking healthcare information. Today, DNA Direct is helping people go one step further by providing individuals with unparalleled access to confidential genetic testing, insight into their personal genetic make-up, expert genetic support and links to resources that can help them lead longer, healthier lives.

As a direct-to-consumer genetic testing company, DNA Direct offers consumers an unprecedented array of genetic tests and pairs each test result with a comprehensive, personalized interpretation. The result is a highly confidential means for people to take a more active role in their health and well being.

"Genetic testing can help us understand who we are and empowers an individual to make informed decisions about health management," says Direct's Medical Director, Katherine Rauen, MD, PhD, DNA. "With just over 2,000 genetic counselors nationwide and even fewer medical geneticists, most people don't have access to genetic testing. DNA Direct is bridging this gap to provide people with a resource to better understand, evaluate and, if they choose, work with their physicians to better manage their health and healthcare decisions."

"DNA Direct provides access to those genetic tests where knowing about your genes can make a big difference, such as when planning a family, selecting a form of birth control or starting hormone replacement therapy," said Ryan Phelan, Founder and CEO, DNA Direct. "It's important to keep in mind that genes are not the sole factor in determining an individual's destiny—family history, lifestyle and environment all play an integral part."

The results of a genetic test can help confirm or rule out a suspected genetic condition or help determine an individual's risk of developing or passing on a genetic disorder.

- Studies estimate that 60,000 to 200,000 people die each year from blood clots. At the high end, this disease kills more people than breast cancer, car accidents and AIDS combined. And 1 in 20 Americans carry a gene, factor V Leiden, which can increase the risk for dangerous blood clots when combined with medical treatments (hormone replacement therapy, birth control pills) or other factors (obesity, smoking, long-haul plane flights). When you know you have genetic propensity for blood clots, you can take action to minimize your risk. (DNA Direct Test at the time this book went to press): Thrombophilia; cost: $380)

- About 35 million people in the U.S.—as many as 1 in 4 people of Irish descent, and 1 in 10 Caucasians—are at risk for a hereditary iron overload disorder that causes a wide variety of symptoms, including chronic fatigue, weakness, joint pain and arthritis. If undetected, iron overload can lead to serious problems, including diabetes, liver and heart disease. But with early detection, effective treatment can stop the progression and even reverse some of the symptoms. (DNA Direct Test: Hemochromatosis; cost at Direct DNA (at the time this book went to press): $199.25)

- About 116 million people worldwide—and up to 1 in 10 Americans—are Alpha-1 carriers. Alpha-1 antitrypsin deficiency is one of the most common genetic disorders worldwide. It is often misdiagnosed, most often as asthma. Early diagnosis can help people at risk take steps to prevent lung and liver disease. A simple genetic test is available for alpha-1 antitrypsin deficiency.

(DNA Direct Test: Alpha-1 Antitrypsin Deficiency; cost at Direct DNA (at the time this book went to press): $330).

DNA Direct currently offers the following genetic tests:

- *Chronic Lung/Liver Disease* (Alpha1-Antitrypsin)
- *Cystic Fibrosis (CFTR)*
- *Hereditary Iron Overload* (Hemochromatosis, HFE)
- *Inherited Blood Clotting Disorders* (Factor V Leiden and Prothrombin)
- *Infertility Panel* (Fragile -X, Cystic Fibrosis, Thrombophilia, Hemochromatosis, Chromosome Analysis, Y Chromosome Deletion)

Ask about DNA Direct's tests for inherited cancer susceptibility. All prices include a Personalized Report that **interprets results** and offers personalized suggestions for lowering risk, and making well-informed decisions about healthcare. Each report also includes information about putting together a healthcare team, and how to approach sharing information with family members and your physician. Test prices (at the time this book went to press) start at $199.25. Due to confidentiality considerations, DNA Direct does not process insurance claims but does provide information and documentation should you choose to submit an insurance claim on your own.

About DNA Direct

San Francisco-based DNA Direct is a personalized genetic testing company focused on consumer education, empowerment and support. With a promise of providing "Your Genes in Context," DNA Direct's mission is to empower individuals with insight into their genetic make-up, including risk factors, preventive measures and action-oriented information to reduce personal risk, coupled with one-on-one support from DNA Direct's genetic experts. All of DNA Direct's services are completely confidential. For more information, go to www.dnadirect.com or call 877.646.0222.

Personalized Genetic Tests Offered

The results of a genetic test can help confirm or rule out a suspected genetic condition or help determine an individual's risk of developing or passing on a genetic disorder. Once a genetic condition is known, preventative and/or treatment choices can often be made. All DNA Direct tests are selected to help people make better health care and lifestyle decisions. DNA Direct currently offers the following genetic tests:

- *Chronic Lung/Liver Disease* (Alpha1-Antitrypsin)
- *Cystic Fibrosis (CFTR)*
- *Hereditary Iron Overload* (Hemochromatosis, HFE)
- *Inherited Blood Clotting Disorders* (Factor V Leiden and Prothrombin)
- *Infertility Panel* (Fragile—X, Cystic Fibrosis, Thrombophilia, Hemochromatosis, Chromosome Analysis, Y Chromosome Deletion)

All prices include a Personalized Report that interprets results and offers personalized suggestions for lowering risk, and making well-informed healthcare decisions. Each report also includes information about putting together a healthcare team, and sharing information with family members and your physician. Due to confidentiality considerations, DNA Direct does not process insurance claims but does provide information and documentation should individuals choose to submit insurance claims on their own.

TEST: INHERITED BLOOD CLOTTING DISORDERS (THROMBOPHILIA)

More than 19 million Americans carry a gene for thrombophilia. If you are one of them, you can take action to prevent dangerous blood clots and live a healthier life. Studies estimate that 60,000 to 200,000 people die each year from blood clots.

At the high end, this disease kills more people than breast cancer, car accidents and AIDS combined. And 1 in 20 Americans carry the gene, factor V Leiden, which can increase the risk for dangerous blood clots when combined with medical treatments (hormone replacement therapy, birth control pills) or other factors (obesity, smoking, long-haul plane flights). When you know you have genetic propensity for blood clots, you can take action to minimize your risk.

Quality Lab Analysis: DNA analysis of the two most common mutations in the factor V and prothrombin genes by a CLIA-certified laboratory.

Quality Lab Analysis:	DNA analysis of the two most common mutations in the factor V and prothrombin genes by a CLIA-certified laboratory.
Home Test Kit:	Cheek Swab
Test Process:	Order a test online and receive a test kit in the mail. Use the painless cheek swab in the privacy of your home

and mail it to our lab in the postage-paid envelope. When the results are ready, we notify you by email. Log on to your secure, password protected account to get your results and Personalized Report online.

Personalized Report: Explains test results and interprets your genes in context, considering age, health, lifestyle, family concerns, preventive steps, resources and much more.

Expert Support: Genetics experts are available to answer questions and provide support
(toll-free 877-646-0222 or expert@dnadirect.com)

Price: $380

TEST: IRON OVERLOAD (HEMOCHROMATOSIS)

Hemochromatosis is an iron overload disorder that can effectively be prevented or treated—but it is often undiagnosed or misdiagnosed. About 35 million people in the U.S.—as many as 1 in 4 people of Irish descent, and 1 in 10 Caucasians—are at risk for a hereditary iron overload disorder that causes a wide variety of symptoms, including chronic fatigue, weakness, joint pain and arthritis. If undetected, iron overload can lead to serious problems, including diabetes, liver and heart disease. But with early detection, effective treatment can stop the progression and even reverse some of the symptoms.

Quality Lab Analysis: DNA analysis of the two most common mutations in the HFE gene by a CLIA-certified laboratory.

Home Test Kit: Cheek Swab

Test Process: Order a test online and receive a test kit in the mail. Use the painless cheek swab in the privacy of your home and mail it to our lab in the postage-paid envelope. When the results are ready, we notify you by email. Log on to your secure, password protected account to get your results and Personalized Report online.

Personalized Report: Explains test results and interprets your genes in context, considering age, health, lifestyle, family history, preventive steps, resources and much more.

Expert Support: Genetics experts are available to answer questions and provide support
(toll-free 877-646-0222 or expert@dnadirect.com)

Price: $199.25

TEST: CHRONIC LUNG/LIVER DISEASE (ALPHA1-ANTITRYPSIN)

Alpha-1 antitrypsin deficiency is one of the most common genetic disorders worldwide. It is often misdiagnosed, most often as asthma. In early stages it can cause breathing difficulties, fatigue, and weakness, and eventually it can lead to chronic obstructive lung disease (COPD), emphysema, and liver failure. Early diagnosis can help people at risk take steps to prevent lung and liver disease. About 116 million people worldwide—and up to 1 in 10 Americans—are Alpha-1 carriers.

Quality Lab Analysis:	DNA analysis of the two most common mutations in the Alpha-1 gene by a CLIA-certified laboratory.
Home Test Kit:	Cheek Swab
Test Process:	Order a test online and receive a test kit in the mail. Use the painless cheek swab in the privacy of your home and mail it to our lab in the postage-paid envelope. When the results are ready, we notify you by email. Log on to your secure, password protected account to get your results and Personalized Report online.
Personalized Report:	Explains test results and interprets your genes in context, considering age, health, lifestyle, family history, preventive steps, resources and much more.
Expert Support:	Genetics experts are available to answer questions and provide support (toll-free 877-646-0222 or expert@dnadirect.com)
Price:	$330

PANEL TEST: INFERTILITY

Infertility Panel:

Tests Included:	Fragile -X, Cystic Fibrosis, Thrombophilia, Hemochromatosis, Chromosome Analysis, Y Chromosome Deletion
Home Test Kit:	Blood sample
Test Process:	Order a test online and receive a test kit in the mail. Visit a nearby clinic affiliate to have a simple, anonymous blood sample taken. Mail your informed consent in the postage-paid envelope to DNA Direct. When the results are ready, we notify you by email. Log on to your secure,

password protected account to get your results and Personalized Report online.

Personalized Report: Explains test results and interprets your genes in context, considering age, health, lifestyle, family concerns, preventive steps, resources and much more.

Expert Support: Genetics experts are available to answer questions and provide support (toll-free 877-646-0222 or expert@dnadirect.com)

Price: male panel $1248.25, female panel $1,191.50

- Prices subject to change without further notice

Other DNA-testing companies online test DNA for ancestry, or molecular anthropology research. Those might be of interest to family historians and genealogists or surname groups seeking a genetic signature of ancestors and descendants related to a common ancestor or particular surname. Some families want to build time capsules that contain not only family history but family medical information for future generations. Some DNA testing companies that are online test for reactions to medicines or foods, such as the speed at which your body metabolizes anesthetic.

Online you'll find numerous companies marketing various DNA tests or kits. Some of these genetic tests are to find out how your body reacts to various dosages of drugs or even foods and skin products. How do you tailor your medicines, foods, cosmetics, anesthetics, dosages, or lifestyles to your genetic signature? Can you find out by genetic tests which type of dental anesthesia you can tolerate and which you're type makes you feel jittery or convulsive? What about tests to find out how your hair tint affects your heart beat? What kinds of tests are out there?

You'll need a consumer's guide to genetic testing kits. Research the various companies online and the studies that include side effects of whatever product or medicine you think you might have to use. Your goal is to safely tailor your environment and lifestyle to your genetic expression or signature.

Consumer's Guide to Genetic Testing

Your DNA, including your ancient ancestry and ethnicity has a lot to do with how your body responds to food, medicine, illness, exercise, and lifestyle, but just how much? And how do you know which DNA kits and gene testing are reliable and recognized?

Learning about DNA to understand and improve your health is now interactive and available to the average consumer, not limited to students and teachers, but to anyone else. In the last few years genealogy buffs, parents, and anyone interested in DNA without a science background took an interest in DNA tests rests that reveal deep maternal and paternal ancestry. Currently consumers with little or no science background are interested in learning about drug metabolism—pharmacogenetics. Referring to the whole human genome that science related to linking pharmacy with genetics is called pharmacogenomics.

How your body metabolizes medicine is as important as how your body metabolizes food. Nutrigenomics is about how your genes respond to food and how to tailor what you eat to your DNA. Consumer DNA interest ranges from forensics and anthropology to nutrition, care giving, family scrap booking and healthcare knowledge. Nurses are becoming more interested in DNA.

The DNA consumer revolution began when media broadcasts revealed to the public that fast computers had revealed the human gene code. Once more TV opened doors. Suddenly, a gap between science and consumers had to be bridged by available interactive education.

A proliferation of products relating to DNA emerged. The internet shows DNA summer day camps for students and teachers. DNA testing companies and books emerged geared to the average consumer. Genealogists tried to interpret DNA for ancestry. People left other non-science-related businesses to open up DNA testing companies for ancestry research, contracting out to university research laboratories to do the DNA testing. Again, opportunities opened doors to the public.

Nutrigenomics product marketers sought those who wanted a diet tailored to their genetic signature. Pharmacogenetics reports customized medicines in order to prevent adverse drug reactions. Pharmacogenomics studies the entire genome in relation to chemicals and drugs, whereas pharmacogenetics researches specific genes and markers to look for adverse drug reactions for individual clients or patients. Finally, DNA testing products emerged offering to tailor skin care products such as creams and cosmetics to your individual genetic signature.

If you've had an interest in learning about how to interpret your DNA test results for ancestry, you now can see the links to understanding how to tailor your food, lifestyle, exercise, medicines, supplements, and skin care products—in fact numerous environmental chemicals—to your genetic expression. It's not only about food anymore or ancestry alone, or medicine.

DNA testing also is about kits sent to you directly or to your physician. It's about tailoring to your DNA skin products, cosmetics and anything you put into or on your body that gets absorbed. It's about what chemicals are in your water and home-grown vegetables.

No science background? Don't worry. There's a DNA summer camp near you, or an educational experience in learning about DNA now available to the average consumer. Educators, scientists, and multimedia producers have teamed up to teach you the wonders of DNA, your genes and your lifestyle.

What's left? Physicians and genetic research scientists need to talk more to each other because most family doctors don't have time to read the proliferation of publications reporting new advances in genetics or other areas of science that directly affect consumers. It looks like it's the consumer's job to bring people together through the media and through consumer's watchdog organizations, professional associations, and support groups. Key words: action and public education about DNA through multimedia and consumer involvement. I highly recommend the DNA Interactive Web site at: http://www.dnalc.org/. Consumers need to know more about how to interpret DNA test results for whatever purpose they seek—tailoring diets or drugs, skin care products, or seeking out ancient family history or ancestral lineages. The science is new enough to have many more applications on the horizon that consumers can digest in the future. What can the average consumer with no science background learn about applications of DNA testing currently? Start with the publications and the interactive DNA learning sites.

You'll soon become familiar with the DNA terminology. The goal is to bridge the gap between science and the consumer, let alone the gap between science and medicine. So you'll have to invite your busy family doctor to join you in creating consumer groups. It'll work fine. Doctors and scientists usually are found conversing together at parties.

The triangle now includes the consumer. If you have children, bring them into the fold. There are now wonderful DNA summer camps. So include your children's teachers. Learning about DNA as a consumer might make you wish you had majored in genetics. Link your beginning self-taught DNA studies to your special field of interest such as your healthcare or your ancestry.

For history buffs, there's always molecular genealogy for family history. History buffs can follow population genetics. Anthropology enthusiasts can read about archaeogenetics. Bring archaeology and DNA together.

Nutrigenomics links DNA research to nutrition for the diet-conscious. Pharmacogenetics helps you to tailor specific medicines to your genes. DNA gets into all walks of life and work. Start with population genetics and physical anthropology if you wish. I like the popular book titled: *The Real Eve*, by Stephen Oppenheimer, Carroll & Graf Publishers, New York, 2003. Or start with nutrition and genetics. First find out what field you like best—nutrition, pharmacy, genealogy, anthropology, or healthcare—and read a book for beginners on DNA related to understanding your particular area of interest, such as nutrition or family history. It's about discoveries.

- Blizzards of discoveries are published monthly in recognized scientific journals found in local medical school libraries open to the public. Only a few consumers ever look at them, and still fewer physicians. Doctors are busy with so many patients and paperwork or bureaucracy. Consumers may not know information is accessible to them. And few can keep up with the proliferation of material in science publications.

- For information, resources, the research network, and references on pharmacogenetics (education) see the Pharmacogenetics and Pharmacogenomics Knowledge Base Web site at: https://preview.pharmgkb.org/resources/education.jsp. As far as education, the Web site features links and articles on the following subjects: What is Pharmacogenetics? Asthma Case Study, CYP2D6 Case Study, The National Institutes of General Medical Sciences (NIGMS), Medicines For You, Minority Pharmacogenomics, The Importance of Genetic Variation in Drug Development, Publications, and News Clippings.

- Click on the Dolan DNA Learning Center at: http://www.dnalc.org/. The Dolan DNA Learning Center at Cold Spring Harbor is entirely devoted to public genetics education. The gene almanac is an online resource that provides timely information about genes in education. The Dolan DNA Learning Center is the world's first science museum and educational facility promoting DNA literacy.

- Dolan's Saturday DNA program is designed to offer children, teens and adults the opportunity to perform hands-on DNA experiments and learn about the latest developments in the biological sciences.

- If you're interested in student "DNA Camps" see the Web site at: http://www.dnalc.org/programs/workshops.html. Student summer day camps have fun with DNA and enzymes and study DNA science or genetic biology. Students and high-school teachers can participate. There are a lot of ways to become involved in learning more on these topics. I wish there were DNA day camps for senior citizens newly retired with time free at last, or for parents, children, and teachers to participate and learn together.

The student summer day camp workshops feature such wonderful learning experiences as the genomic biology and PCR workshop. This new workshop is based on lab and computer technology developed at the DNALC in the past year. The workshop focuses on the use of the polymerase chain reaction (PCR) to analyze the genetic complement (genome) of humans and plants. DNA educational centers bridge gaps between scientists and communicators.

Many physicians have not yet been trained in nutritional genomics or in phar-macogenetics—how to correctly interpret a DNA test for consumers. Who advises consumers how to tailor their food or drugs to their genes in ways that consumers can immediately use? Who instructs them how to make time capsules out of their ancestry from DNA reports?

For the time being, it's the bioscience journalist who acts as a communicator, the liaison, the publicist, the broadcaster, the bearer of news, the turner of com-plex terms into plain language, the reporter and the publisher, showing con-sumers, physicians, and scientists how to bridge the gap between science and healthcare.

Who acts as the middle person between genetics and medicine or between nutrition and healthcare? Who bridges the gap between the dietician and the geneticist? For now, it's the media, the science writer writing for the mass media or an audience of general readers—consumers like you and I. Who should join the science media team? Check out consumer watchdog groups, concerned physicians, genetics researchers—scientists, DNA testing companies, and bio-science publishers.

Instead of worrying about physician apathy or consumers turning to alterna-tive medicine, let's turn to scientific knowledge available to all consumers if you know where to look and what is accessible. If you want to take charge over how your body responds to food or medicine or lifestyle changes, you need to take control by finding out how your genes respond to what you put into your body from what you eat to the drugs you take to the chemicals in your environment.

Has a local or national newspaper reported on rocket fuel or other specific chemicals in your water supply that went into your home-grown vegetables that made your thyroid go wild, find out what research is being done on the situation. Or if your body responds to various foods in certain ways or various drugs in other ways, you can take control by learning what new advances are available to you. Check out what is credible and what works for you. Minorities may have genes that respond differently to various dosages of med-icines. Check out the Web site for research on minority pharmacogenetics at: <http://www.sph.uth.tmc.edu:8057/gdr/default.htm>.   The   Minority Pharmacogenetics website is devoted to issues of minorities, populations and pharmacogenomics.

Have you ever met a doctor who keeps up with all the latest advances? Who has time? Consumers do. Look at the breakthroughs in the journals published monthly. Why worry that medical discoveries aren't being delivered fast enough to patients or clients if you can see what's happening in the journals?

Consumers need to form watchdog groups and to link up with the media. You need to become involved in accessing scientific pioneers. As a journalist, my job is to convey information to the public to bridge the communication gap. As a consumer, your job is to take care of your body. Nobody should walk in medical or nutritional ignorance when the information you might need "is out there." You don't need any science degree or license to read public information. Let's all bridge the communication gap between consumers, scientists, and physicians.

Consumers want applied knowledge. Here's where to start. On the Web, look at: http://www.nigms.nih.gov/funding/medforyou.html. It's the page for The National Institutes of General Medical Sciences (NIGMS). It's the home page for the National Institute of General Medical Sciences, a component of the National Institutes of Health, the principle biomedical research agency of the United States Government. "NIGMS supports basic biomedical research that is not targeted to specific diseases, but that increases understanding of life processes and lays the foundation for advances in disease diagnosis, treatment, and prevention," according to the Pharmacogenetics and Pharmactogenomics Knowledge Base at: http://www.nigms.nih.gov/funding/medforyou.html.

If your doctor hasn't the time to take advantage of current treatment findings, you as a consumer can read what your physician may not get to read for a while. Picture one future fantastic scenario regarding DNA testing where spouses are chosen based on DNA reports. If this scenario sounds too bizarre, then visualize choosing foods based on DNA reports. That sounds credible. The point made here is that you could help to bridge the gap between research and conventional medicine. You and I have our work cut out for us, speaking as a consumer and as a journalist who loves reading scientific articles.

The scene at the "speed dating" table opens with a young woman waving her latest DNA test result under the nose of her blind date. "I'll show you mine, if you'll show me yours," she says, smiling. The fellow opens his DNA test result folder or database. They exchange DNA test result printouts and interpretations. "Hmm…regarding ancestry," he says, "Looks like we're both members of the same mtDNA matrilineal clan."

That could be haplogroup H, L, M, or with whatever worldwide mtDNA haplogroup letter or matrilineal 'clan' they match. "Now let's look at your specific genetic markers and genes tested for adverse reactions to this list of medicines or foods or…" She gazes up at him smiling. "I like your lack of risk for diseases," he says. "And I like the way your gene mutations put you at risk for all these inheritable diseases," she answers.

"Do you also have any inheritable real estate and cash? I'd like to be beneficiary." He looks at her askance and holds up a little green bottle. "With this gene equalizer, my risk is greatly lowered." They exchange DNA printouts once more and move to different tables to begin another Dating by DNA interview.

Would you consider a science fiction version of "blind dating by DNA?" Maybe, but consumers want practical results from DNA testing that they can apply to real-life situations. What kind of personalized medicine can consumers find today regarding genetic testing? How many ways can you use DNA tests? Tailoring your food, customizing your medicines by avoiding adverse drug reactions, looking at your ancient ancestry, family history, or genealogy by DNA through "molecular genetics" and perhaps, choosing your spouse by DNA?

Genetic screening of couples hoping to marry or couples seeking answers to fertility questions have been screened for inheritable diseases in several countries. How many ways can you market DNA tests? For what purposes can you use DNA tests? Who will review the products? Consumers need a guide to genetic testing kits that can be sold directly to the public and also to physicians and other healthcare providers.

Personalized Medicine from DNA Testing Companies

How do consumers or consumer's watchdog groups regulate doctors' services? Are DNA test kits sold to consumers really doctor's services or are they medical devices? Consumers want their healthcare and nutrition tailored to their individual genetic signatures, and they want it to be affordable and available to everyone. The FDA regulates medical devices, not physician's services. Where does a DNA kit sent directly to consumers fit into a definition? Scientists and physicians study haplotypes when they map complex-disease genes. Genetic researchers look at the abundance of single-nucleotide polymorphisms (SNPs). They use terms such as "single-locus analyses."

Consumers want those terms translated into plain language by bioscience communicators, since most scientists and physicians are too busy to continuously write about genes for the public. That's why public education programs about DNA exist, including the summer day camps for students and teachers. We need the training programs and camps also for parents—for entire families from great grandma and grandpa to elementary school children and teens.

When it comes to studying how your genes respond to food or drugs, scientists avoid analyses techniques with limited power and instead focus on economical alternatives to molecular-haplotyping methods. So you, as a consumer, presumably with little or no science background, are in a position to learn about your own genes and about DNA in general.

You can start with some of the DNA public education learning programs open to anyone. Since the gene hunters began to explore the entire human genome, they opened a door to the public for knowledge accessible to all. At first consumers were interested in learning how to interpret their DNA test for ancestry and family history. Next, consumers wanted to know how to tailor their drugs and food to their genes—their genetic expression. Finally, consumers found they could customize skin care products to their DNA reports as well.

Consumers ask important questions. What's waiting for you in a DNA kit that will be valuable to your health? How will you understand and apply the scientific reports to your daily lifestyle? How do you find out whether the various DNA testing companies are credible and recognized by which group? Who are the watchdogs here? Who are the experts? What do you do with the information you receive after a DNA test? Should you test for deep ancestry, adverse response to drugs, or tailoring your food to your DNA? How do you apply the information in a practical way?

Should the consumer only deal with companies that sell their DNA test kits to physicians and similar healthcare professions such as dieticians and genetics counselors? Or should the average consumer buy a DNA testing kit directly from a company that also markets to consumers, bypassing physicians? What do you think as a consumer? Which stance are you taking? For resources and articles, see the Web site at: http://syndromexmenu.tripod.com.

What happens when a DNA testing company sells its DNA tests or kits to companies that turn around and sell personalized nutritional or cosmetics products so that consumers can buy skin products or nutritional supplements customized to their genetic signatures? Is this good for consumers? What do you think? I like DNA testing. The interpretation of the tests is tricky. Results can have a lot more than one interpretation, even for physicians and scientists. So how does the consumer learn to screen the screeners?

Should a company tell consumers which specific genes are tested? Some companies do and others don't. How do you know whether the dose of vitamins you take is beneficial or harmful? Do you need to cut back or add more? What can DNA testing do for you, the consumer, presumably starting with no science background? As a bioscience journalist, I'm not taking sides here, but I really like the variety of DNA tests.

Some types of genetic test kits are sold directly to the public, and others are marketed only to physicians and similar healthcare professionals. From the consumer's point of view, there is always the question of whether the tests are needed and if they are, how accurate and valuable are the tests, and who is trained and experienced enough to interpret the answers?

If you're going to take a DNA test, it could be for ancestry, for nutrition planning, or to see whether any prescribed or over-the-counter drug, chemical, supplement, nutraceutical, food, or herb you take will have adverse effects on your body. For years you could test for allergies to some substances and foods, some chemicals in the environment, but now there's genetic testing.

Specific genes are tested for risk or reaction. The type of consumer most likely to order a genetic test for drug response or a "pharmacogenetic test" would be an individual with medical conditions taking several drugs and concerned how his or her body handled the mix of medicines, food, and lifestyle. Each person has his or her own genetic signature.

You rinse your mouth with a type of mouthwash and send the contents in a small tube to a laboratory, hospital, office, or company to be analyzed. Or you swab the inside of your cheek with a felt tip and send the swab to a hospital or genetic testing company so your DNA—specific genetic markers—can be analyzed.

In a few weeks, you get a report. The genetic testing company looks at specific genes and markers. If you're concerned about drugs, you want to know how slowly your body is breaking down any of the drugs you take or might take in the future. You don't want to gulp down a prescription or over-the-counter drug and have it build up in your body to the point you land in the emergency room of a hospital. The whole point of a genetic test for adverse drug reactions is to alert your physician to adjust the dosage of your medicine or change the type of medicine.

On one side, the consumer sees the physician and scientist diagnosing rare diseases by looking at particular genes. On the other, the consumer wants information on how genes work. Firms that sell gene tests directly to consumers need to fill an education gap. Certain tests can be sold directly to consumers, such as DNA testing for ancestry, genealogy, family, oral history, DNA matches, and surname projects where people with the same or similar last names are matched by DNA to see whether there's a relationship in former times.

What DNA testing companies can do for the consumer is to widely teach the consumer about population genetics—the peopling of the world. How about for disease? Genetic disease specialists have been in charge of this new science. Lately, companies that test DNA now market directly to consumers as well as to their physicians. Here's a chance to educate consumers as well as physicians in everything they need to know about their genes. Physicians want to know how to interpret DNA tests for disease markers. Consumers want this information directly. So there needs to be a level for education for both physician and consumer.

If a DNA testing firm markets directly to the consumer, the test should be interpreted for the consumer and the physician. Consumers are paying to learn what medications to avoid. Allergists usually told people what foods to avoid. What consumers want is to know what foods, vitamins, minerals, supplements, skin creams, herbs, medicines, and other nutraceuticals will work best with their individual genetic signatures.

Who will teach consumers how to interpret genetic test results? Who trains most physicians presently? Either the DNA testing companies must educate the consumer, or the consumer as an autodidact, must teach himself from reliable sources.

Today anyone with a genealogy hobby an open a DNA testing company and contract out to a laboratory in a university to test DNA for clients. When it comes to test DNA for diseases or drug reactions, it's different than sending a printout regarding the client's ancient general ancestry such as the results of a DNA test for mtDNA (matrilineal ancestry) or Y-chromosome (patrilineal ancestry) in the deep past. Those tests are general and would be of interest to people matching ancestors or learning about population genetics and ancient migrations.

When it comes to tailoring food or drugs to your genotype, how far can DNA testing companies bypass the genetic disease specialists and market directly to the consumer? The answer is as far as it takes to teach the consumer about his or her own genetic expression. When you look for a DNA testing company, ask yourself whether the company diagnoses diseases? Does the company help you choose your medicines, food, or cosmetics according to your genetic signature? Or does the company work with your physician and you. Does the company pass you over entirely and only send the results to your personal physician?

Look at the marketing efforts of the company. Investigate gene research for yourself by the many articles available online and in the medical libraries and popular magazines that go to physicians. If you buy a test, is it affordable? Do you need the particular DNA test?

If one of your relatives has a specific condition you might have inherited that will show symptoms when you reach a certain age or presently, you need to know what you can do to delay or prevent the situation. You need to know that the results of DNA testing are for a particular purpose, such as testing adverse reactions of your body to certain prescription drugs. Find out the value of the tests from reliable sources. If you start with your personal physician, make sure he or she can correctly interpret a genetics test. Some physicians can't because they were never trained to do so.

Consult the various professional associations for referrals to genetic disease specialists rather than rely on a generalist when it comes to interpreting your test while you learn how to interpret your tests yourself. The purpose is to make sure your physician's interpretation and your interpretation agree. If you have any doubt, you need more information and a second opinion.

What you want to avoid is confusion. Are the tests available today reliable? Find out from several opinions of specialists. To reach these specialists, the professional associations for the various genetic disease specialists would be of help as would the publications. You can talk to the research labs at universities specializing in genetic testing. The institutes are online and have their own Web sites.

Talk to federal health officials about what's on the consumer market in your country and in other countries. Some people send their DNA swabs to companies and/or labs in other countries. Currently genetic tests are sold without a special 'watch' organization that reviews them. So look at any publications put out by the U.S. Food and Drug Administration (FDA). The FDA wants consumers to become more involved in their own food safety and security monitoring. Keep a folder on DNA testing company marketing claims and check them out.

Companies can tell you which mix of vitamins works best or what food to eat based on genetic testing and/or health questionnaires. For example, check out GeneLink Inc., New Jersey. Their Web site is at: http://www.bankdna.com/breakthrough_profiling.html.

According to an investment Web site called Multex, listed at: http://biz.yahoo.com/p/g/gnlk.ob.html, GeneLink Inc. is described as a bioscience company that offers the safe collection and preservation of a family's DNA material. It's for later use by the family. The collection is used to identify and potentially prevent inherited diseases.

GeneLink has created a new methodology for single nucleotide polymorphisms (SNPs)-based on genetic profiling. The Company plans to license these proprietary assessments to companies that manufacture or market to the nutraceutical, personal care, skin care, and weight-loss industries.

"GeneLink's operations can be divided into two segments, the biosciences business, which includes three SNP-based, proprietary genetic indicator tests, and DNA Banking, which involves the use of its proprietary DNA Collection Kit." Contact GeneLink at: 100 S. Thurlow Street, Margate, NJ 08402. See the Web site at: http://biz.yahoo.com/p/g/gnlk.ob.html.

GeneLink also offers gene testing for skin care products. According to a March 6, 2003 media release posted at GeneLink's "In the News" Web page at: http://www.bankdna.com/news_articles/03_06_03.html, GeneLink, Inc. (OTCBB:GNLK) "entered into a collaborative agreement with DNAPrint Genomics, Inc. (OTCBB:DNAP) whereby the companies will combine certain scientific and intellectual property resources to develop and market 'next generation' genetic profile tests to the $100 Billion plus personal care and cosmetics industry." Further details were not disclosed.

"GeneLink invented the first genetically-designed patentable DNA test for customized skin-care products, and DNAPrint brings its ultra-high throughput genotype capability and ADMIXMAP platform to the partnership. The companies anticipate screening millions of candidate markers to broaden proprietary product offerings. Tests are designed to assess genetic risks for certain skin and nutritional deficiencies and provide a basis for recommending formulations that have been specifically designed to compensate for these deficiencies."

I like this idea. I'm allergic to hair tint and aloe vera, and it would b wonderful to find skin care products that didn't turn my skin red and make it itch. Think of all the allergy warnings and patch tests on hair products. If everyone walked into a beauty salon with a list of products that can be safely put on the scalp or other skin without an adverse response, that list would be my definition of comfort. Also, check out GeneLink's test which tells clients which mix of vitamins is appropriate for an individual's genes without getting an adverse reaction from the vitamin combination. I know certain supplements over-stimulate my thyroid. I'd love to have these kinds of tests.

How about you? Still, you need to do your homework on the usefulness of the tests or the claims. Perhaps you need to deal with a company in another country. Sciona Ltd. in England gives nutritional advice based on your DNA and a questionnaire related to your health. *The company sells tests only through doctors and dieticians.* How do you know which defect is associated with any specific gene when the gene is defective? With so many interpretations, consumers can become confused from test results. Sometimes scientists in various companies don't know which results are accurate predictions. That's why consumer watchdog groups are necessary.

The only problem is that the average consumer usually can't afford to hire genetics counselors unless they have a specific genetic disease. If you have a reduced ability to process something, it's not a disease, but unless you take action, your body could suffer in other ways resulting from the reduced ability to process an essential nutrient from your diet that your body needs to work with other processes. It's like a chain reaction.

That's why DNA testing is helpful. At the same time, you can't assume some people need more of one vitamin just because their body processes a nutrient at a reduced rate. The science is still very new. A lot of data is still in the works. You don't know whether certain genetic profiles need special diets. Consumers want to see rare clinical data. Consumers most of all want to know the value of what the DNA tests predict. And no one wants to take a test and then worry for a decade.

What consumers want are not only tests of prescription drugs and food as to whether adverse reactions happen with individuals based on their genetic testing, but personalized anti-aging formulas, cosmetics, creams, and other products customized to the individual's genetic markers are needed.

These tests must be reliable, consumers say. Feedback is helpful. Customer reviews of the companies are needed. Who will publish customer reviews of the products and the DNA testing firms? These consumer reviews could also include input from scientists and physicians. Physicians should take the DNA testing themselves after they are properly trained to interpret the tests before looking at their patient's results.

Nutritionists and dieticians show concern that medical schools only give very brief and shallow courses in nutrition to graduating physicians. What about a course in interpreting genetics tests? Will this be left to naturopaths and homeopaths? Or can medical schools include courses in DNA test interpretation to physicians other than genetic disease specialists? Healthcare consumers should ask for DNA testing from their HMOs before taking prescribed medicines. Will insurance companies pay for testing?

Look at the various DNA testing companies. Also look at health screening companies. One would be HealthcheckUSA, San Antonio, Texas for example, sells a mail-order test for iron buildup in the blood known as hereditary hemochromatosis. Results go to the consumer. If you need a test for cystic fibrosis or a blood clotting disorder known as factor V Leiden, check out this company. Their Web site is at: http://www.healthcheckusa.com/media.html, or you can write to them at: *HealthcheckUSA*, 8700 Crownhill Rd., Suite 110, San Antonio, TX 78209.

Practicing physicians started HealthCheck USA in 1987 to provide health awareness screening to customers throughout the USA. The tests provided to their customers are the same as those ordered by physicians across the country. Many physicians refer their patients to Healthcheck USA. Since 1987, HealthCheck USA has provided over 500,000 health awareness screening tests to satisfied customers nationwide.

The company is associated with the country's major fully accredited medical reference laboratories, to ensure quality, accurate test results. HealthcheckUSA has partnered with Virtual Medical Group, Inc., to offer physician interpretation of results. According to HealthcheckUSA's Web site, "You can have your results reviewed and interpreted by a Board Certified Physician. By selecting the "Physician Interpretation of Results" option, you will be mailed instructions with the hard copy of your results. These instructions will give you a toll free number along with your username and password to access your interpretation 72 hours after your blood draw. This process is completely confidential, private, and secure."

Here the consumer has the best of both worlds. What tests are provided? Check out the list of tests provided at the Web site: http://www.healthcheckusa. com/testsweoffer.php.

When any company does health screening, find out whether it is DNA testing, blood testing, comprehensive tests, or whether you are sent test kits such as for colon cancer screening, prothrombin (factor KII) DNA test, cystic fibrosis (DNA test), Factor V R2 (DNA test) or other. Are the results sent back to you directly as a consumer? Or do you purchase additional services such as a physician's interpretation of the results?

What consumers want are genetic tests for metabolism and health. Doctors used genetic testing when patients were concerned about diagnosing inherited diseases. Today, the general consumer of healthcare and healthcare alternative medicine wants genetic testing for general healthcare in the absence of a specific disease. Consumers want to know how to handle the risks they might have inherited to delay or prevent what happened to their grandparents. Also parents of children and couples worried about fertility issues also want these types of tests. Genetic testing shouldn't be used to screen people out of insurance, employment, or anything else.

Health screening should be focused on matching people to the best possible foods, nutraceuticals, and medicines when and if needed. It should be an inclusive not an exclusive process. Like personnel departments that focus on screening out applicants, genetic testing should not be used to screen people out or to exclude based on genetic risks. Instead, it should be used to draw people into learning about taking responsibility for their own health habits such as choosing the right foods. It's all about choice, like the science of nutrition.

Genetic tests were used on people who suffered from rare genetic disease. Consumers are worried about claims by companies that sell DNA tests to the public. Presently, consumers are asking the FDA to review tests before they are sold to the public or to physicians. The FDA reviews drugs and other medical appliances, why not DNA tests or other health screening tests sold to consumers? Should the government be reviewing these tests?

What do you think? Or should the tests be monitored by the companies offering them? Or should the approach be to the tests similar to vitamins and minerals found in health food stores? What side will you take? Do you have enough information to even begin to take sides? Who runs and regulates the DNA testing companies that may or may not be headed by physicians and geneticists?

Testing DNA for ancestry would not have the same impact on someone's health as testing DNA for a specific disease marker. Still, the people doing the testing should have the same qualifications. What about the people doing the interpreting? What stance do you take? Then there's the question of privacy which is essential.

If you're testing for DNA ancestry, you might want to meet your DNA match to correspond with online. If you're testing for a disease marker, you want privacy. You may want to join a support group of families with similar DNA markers for the specific risk or disease you've inherited. You want meetings held in a hospital or some other private, medical setting. Personal issues come up.

Research the various associations of physicians, such as the American Academy of Family Physicians and other similar groups. You can find opinions there. You can bring in lawyers who want to make sure laws are put into effect to keep employers and insurers from using your results to terminate your job or kick you off of health or life insurance plans if your genes put you at risk.

Set up groups made up of advisories of experts that include consumer groups. What consumers with no science background can do is to work with the US Department of Health and Human Services to monitor various panels of experts. Some people want regulations to change. Others don't. There are hundreds of groups out there who advise the US Dept. of Health on what policies they 'should' adopt.

Consumers ask for reviews. Experts ask for reviews. Consumers don't want their vitamins taken away from health food stores. In the midst of it all are the wonderful DNA tests. Talk to pharmacists as well. If you're having adverse reactions to drugs, you eagerly want a DNA test you can take at home as a consumer. What I like about Genelex Corporation's drug metabolism test is that the test can tell you whether your body is taking too long to break down the drugs you're consuming. Consumers need that kind of calmness that comes from knowing personal physicians aren't prescribing too much of what you may or may not need. Maybe you're worrying about your pharmacist giving you the wrong medicine or dosage. Whatever you're concern, a home DNA test is a tool for consumers.

Monitoring your own health is your responsibility, not merely your doctor's. You can get DNA tests sent to your home or scans from clinics. Prescription drugs are available on the Internet. How your body will metabolize what you put into it is important. Are you becoming your own doctor? Is the average consumer becoming more knowledgeable? Or is it more accurate to say most people haven't an inkling of what DNA is?

Pharamcogenetics and nutrigenomics offer tools to consumers. The movement is towards taking charge of your own healthcare. Are doctors worried consumers are taking money away from them? Do tests create more problems than they solve? What happens when scans or other types of tests show non-existent problems?

Research what comes out of the National Institutes of Health. Consumers want to know what the results of their tests mean and how they can apply the information in practical ways. Who interprets the tests? Who is reviewing genetic tests sent directly to consumers and physicians? Right now, it's the consumer's 'job' to ask these questions. If you don't know what vitamins to take, perhaps you need a DNA test to tell you what vitamins work best with your individual genes.

DNA tests seek out mutations in the genes. If a mutation is only remotely associated with a risk, do you ignore it or customize your food and vitamins to the mutation that is only remotely connected to the risk? What action do you take as a consumer? You talk to a physician who knows about genes and your particular risk or you go to a genetics counselor. If you have certain forms of a gene that results in cancer of a certain area of your body by a certain age, you take action right away. Some mutations are associated with disease and some are not, such as certain ancestry markers.

Some genes account for only a tiny percentage of certain cancers. Not everyone needs to be tested. If you have a family reason to be tested, then get tested. If one of your siblings or parents has an inheritable disease, get tested. You can check out Myriad Genetics based in Utah regarding their breast and ovarian cancer tests, available only through doctors. Their Web site is at: http://www.myriad.com/. Or contact them at: Myriad Genetic Laboratories, Inc. | 320 Wakara Way, SLC UT 84108–1214

The Controversy over Whether Genetic Tests should be Sold to the Public

Professionals working in molecular genetics may be divided among those who think genetic tests should be sold to the general consumer and those who think they should not. The professionals who think genetic tests should not be sold to the public may underestimate the intelligence of the public's drive to learn as much as possible about their own genes—the DNA, ancestry, health response to medicine and chemicals in their environment, their response to prescription and over-the-counter drugs, and their response to food, nutraceuticals and other supplements.

Is genetic testing too complex for the average consumer to understand? Would the subject of genetic testing interest the average reader or consumer?

Is the average consumer someone who says "it's way over my head," or "my eyes are glazing over" when you mention anything scientific? Or is the average consumer an individual who wants to learn as much as possible about his or her own DNA, health, ancestry, and genetic response to food?

Most consumers only need to be told that more than a hundred mutations can cause a specific disorder or disease. Average consumers can understand that. Those who underestimate the intelligence and desire to learn of an individual about his or her own health or the health of children and parents usually are the ones who are first to speak out in censorship of a consumer's right to learn all that is possible to learn at the moment about his own genes.

When a consumer is told that negative results don't always signal health, he or she is intelligent to understand that plain English or any language statement. It's a learning process. Some genetics companies are in direct marketing. Some test

DNA only for ancestry. Other genetics companies test for genetic responses to drugs or for various genetic health risks that can be helped by changes in diet. The aim of these companies is cooperation. That means cooperation between patient, physician, genetics counselor, dietician or nutritionist and anyone else involved in the healthcare team working with the patient.

In fact in genetics testing, patients are really clients seeking information, feedback, and recommendations for changes in lifestyle and diet. In drug response genetic testing, the client wants to know how his or her body metabolizes the prescription or over-the-counter medicines used. The whole idea of genetic testing is to bring the healthcare team closer to the healthcare consumer. Instead of a one-size-fits all attitude with drugs, foods, or nutraceuticals, or the usual five to fifteen minute consultation with a doctor, the consumer can have the chance to learn everything publicly available about how his or her genes respond to food, drugs, chemicals in the environment, or lifestyle changes.

If a genetics testing company markets cancer tests, it should have the responsibility to let the patient know that the tests are meant for specific people with specific familial cancers and not for the entire consumer population. When a genetics company takes a family history, it opens doors to the individual not only to explore a familial inherited disease or risk, but the entire history and ancestry of the person's family and the DNA of the family members.

Individuals need to learn that there could be more than one gene involved. So teaching consumers about their DNA and genes is important. Classes could be springing up to train people what to expect before they undergo testing. It's a matter of learning and teaching. This is one more way to make use of retired professionals and other scientists and physicians or genetics counselors working in molecular genetics—helping consumers learn what they can expect from testing.

Consumers need to learn about how important it is to sequence certain genes from many family members. Consumers need to get in touch with affected family members and form a support group for DNA testing, perhaps creating a time capsule for future generations with genetic information resulting from testing.

Most consumers go to their family doctors first. Yet how many family physicians are interested in, let alone trained in molecular genetics? Not so many. Most physicians may not interpret a genetic test correctly because they haven't been trained to do so. In may be that the consumer is the first person to request training be set up to show physicians how to interpret genetic tests, especially for such diseases as cancer. Consumers have more power as a group. So consumers need to become involved, work together as an organization, and make sure not only the physicians are trained, but also themselves as consumers of genetic testing. Perhaps the physician and consumer can learn together in groups set up for both, where at a point, physician and consumer meet together. Will this present the physician differently in the eyes of the patient? Not really. The science is new enough so that consumer and patient could learn together to unravel the mysteries of genetics not unlike checking the clues in a mystery novel.

Consumers need to read more medical journals such as the New England Journal of Medicine. Spend some time in the library of your local medical school reading about how physicians interpret genetic testing. Look at surveys. As of now, not too many general consumers from the public at large even know what DNA is. So you have to educate yourself, perhaps as a new hobby. First find out what DNA is. Look it up in the dictionary.

Then start reading magazine articles about genetic testing. Look on the Web at the testing companies. Then you can graduate to reading articles in medical journals. The gap between the physician and the consumer needs to be narrowed at least when it comes to your own DNA and genetic testing for the things consumers put into their body such as food and prescribed or over-the-counter medicines, supplements such as herbs, and other nutraceuticals.

Everyone talks about the consumer's consent to testing. The problem is that the consumer needs to be given information. If you're going to eat 'smarter' you have to become informed first. If you have an inheritable risk or disease, you need to understand everything you can find that is publicly accessible about the risk, the disease, or the genes involved. Material is online, but is it credible? There are always the articles in medical journals, but can you understand the terminology? If not, look up the terms in glossaries and dictionaries. Make a list of terms and learn how to make the journal articles understandable in plain language.

Think about risk for a moment. Your risk could change. How are you going to receive the information from genetic testing? What are you going to do about it as far as changing your lifestyle, diet, or medicines? If you are concerned how your family might react to genetic testing, ask them whether they would change their food choices or other lifestyle changes based on the information. You can always keep the information private, but it could save the lives of family members to get tested and to change what can be changed, such as food choices or exercise routines.

Most consumers worry more about discrimination in employment and health insurance due to companies finding out their genetic risks. Privacy must be kept, and information only given to the consumer of the testing, not his employer or health insurance company. It's nobody's business but your own as far as your genetic information. So, measures to keep out strangers from using your genes against you must be in order. That's why numbers instead of names work better with testing.

The big issue is accuracy. If so many physicians cannot correctly interpret a genetic test and advise their patients, more training is needed for the physicians and the patients. It's a case of whose watching the watchers. Who is going to review the genetic testing itself as to accuracy? What if the tests are not accurate? Right now nobody is reviewing the testing companies other than themselves. Nobody is reporting directly to the consumer after checking the accuracy of the genetic tests. And nobody is reporting directly to the physician with that same information.

If you're going to get tested, at least learn as much as most professional genetic counselors know about interpreting your tests. It can be done without going back to school for a graduate degree in molecular genetics. The information is available to the public from libraries, the Internet, databases, and medical school libraries, journals, and professional articles. Many are on the Web in PDF files. Subscribe to the journals or read them in libraries and learn how to interpret your own tests. Then form a consumer's group to watch the watchers. Learn how to check the accuracy of tests done by the testing companies.

You have to become involved in your own healthcare and nutrition. Take charge and take responsibility. Consumers can't be passive. You won't know how your body responds to food or medicine or lifestyle changes until symptoms appear. Start by looking at the health of your family members and realizing what is inheritable, and what you can do to help yourself if you've inherited what they have or will get.

The first step for consumers is to start learning about DNA and genetic testing just as they have learned about genealogy and family history. Classes online or in adult education can be set up as well as support groups and organizations of consumers. The second step is to form a group to review the accuracy of information that comes with your genetic tests. Invite physicians and other healthcare professionals to join with consumers and become a team.

Don't let separation between those with scientific knowledge and those without become a barrier to reviewing accuracy of information. When genetics-trained professionals band together to review the accuracy of information provided with genetic testing, the group usually becomes made up only of professionals. When consumers group together, they include professionals as well as consumers.

So consumers need to create a group to review the accuracy of information that comes with genetic tests. And that same group needs to make sure education exists for consumers. You need to set up classes to train consumers in how to understand the results of their genetic testing and how to review the accuracy of the information given along with the genetic tests.

If trained physicians can't correctly interpret a genetic test for their patients in certain cases, it's time for consumers to take charge of their own healthcare education. Okay, you can't do surgery on yourself, but you can learn to read the information provided with genetic tests.

Learn also to question the accuracy of that information you've read in medical journals and other publications. Consumers can read not only the medical journal articles usually found in medical school and university libraries open to the public, publications such as the *New England Journal of Medicine*, but also some of the more popular articles in magazines that go to physicians such as *Physician's Weekly*.

All this autodidact education can be achieved with consumers involvement and support groups if people are interested enough to involve a wide range of members or participants. Genetic training should be available to everyone equally and widely available through the internet, through senior centers, classrooms focused on adult education, through hospitals and HMO programs, and through the genetic testing companies.

In the magazine, *Physician's Weekly*, October 7, 2002, Vol. XIX, No. 38, the article in Point/Counterpoint, titled, *"Should genetic tests be sold directly to the public?"* featured Howard Coleman, CEO, Genelex Corp., Redmond, Washington and Kimberly A. Quaid, PhD,

Professor of Clinical, Medical, and Molecular Genetics, Clinical Psychiatry, and Clinical Medicine, Indiana University School of Medicine. Coleman's response was yes, and Quaid's response was no. See the article, copyrighted 2002 by *Physician's Weekly*, reprinted below with permission.

Should genetic tests be sold directly to the public?

Howard Coleman, CEO, Genelex Corp., Redmond, Washington.

YES Every person has the right to know his or her genetic information, and the right not to share it. People have legitimate privacy concerns about their genetic information being loose in the medical records system, fearing for their jobs or insurance if it gets into the wrong hands. Physicians are also concerned, and don't want to risk compromising a patient's privacy. This contributes to their reluctance to order genetic tests.

There are compelling reasons for people to obtain reliable genetic information, whether they go through their doctors or not. According to a 1998 JAMA article, more than 100,000 deaths occur annually due to adverse drug reactions, along with an additional 2.2 million serious events that require hospital stays. These are not medical mishaps, as they occur within the labeled use of drugs.

When physicians begin to learn the genotype of their patients they will begin to solve this problem. The practice of their clinical art will be improved because in many instances the genotype of their patient trumps the many other characteristics they do know.

Despite the facts that science has known for the past half century that people react differently to drugs, doctors have been unable to put genetic testing into practice for the benefit of their patients. Doctors lack sufficient training in pharmacogenetics and drug metabolism. For example, most doctors don't know that genotyping for Coumadin metabolism is available, and that it will help patients avoid adverse reactions with this drug.

Adverse drug reactions kill many people in the U.S., but the threat goes largely unrecognized. Making gene tests available directly to patients not only provides a valuable service, but helps push the medical community into the 21st century era of personalized and evidence-based medicine.

Kimberly A. Quaid, PhD, Professor of Clinical, Medical, and Molecular Genetics, Clinical Psychiatry, and Clinical Medicine Indiana University School of Medicine

NO No. Genetic testing is far too complex for lay people to tackle on their own. For example, more than 100 mutations can cause cystic fibrosis, and most genetic tests only cover a small subset of these. But most lay people don't understand that negative results are not necessarily a clean bill of health.

The announcement last spring that Myriad Genetics would direct market cancer tests was particularly troubling, because such tests are only appropriate for a small number of individuals with certain familial cancers. The complex protocol includes taking a detailed family history, then finding and sequencing the gene from affected relatives (and there may be more than one gene).

Individuals who hear about such tests might approach their family physicians, but research shows that many are not trained in genetics. A paper in the NEJM, which looked at physicians ordering a test for a particular cancer, found that one third of these physicians interpreted the test incorrectly. One can assume that if physicians have trouble interpreting the results, patients will fare far worse. One survey found that fewer than 26% of Americans know what DNA is.

Geneticists believe testing should be preceded by informed consent. For consent to be informed, the patient must understand the disorder for which they are being tested, their current risk, how their risk might change as a result of testing, the ramifications of their being tested for their families and spouses, and the possibility of discrimination should third parties get their hands on this information.

Finally, no mechanism exists to review the accuracy of information provided with genetic tests to either health-care professionals or consumers. Individuals who get tested without professional counseling may buy trouble with their test results.

In our recent email interview of August 19, 2003, Howard Coleman added, ""I agree with Dr. Quaid when the testing concerns the grave medical conditions caused by genetic disease and we don't offer those tests to the general public. The testing we do provide can help both the physician and the individual understand their ability to metabolize drugs which can help to prevent adverse drug reactions and how to optimize their diet."

Scientists and Physicians Comment on Pharmacogenetics

Why would the average consumer of health care want to have drug reaction testing, known as pharmacogenetic testing? The field is new, and still emerging. According to (reprinted with permission) Genelex's "Health and DNA" Web site (copyright 2003) at: http://www.healthanddna.com/, "The relatively new and emerging fields of pharmacogenetics studies how differences in individual genetic makeup affect the processing of drugs. We have known for about a half-century that individuals respond to the same drug and dosage in very different ways because of genetic variations called polymorphisms.

Research shows that of all the clinical factors such as age, sex, weight, general health and liver function that alter a patient's response to drugs; genetic factors are the most important. Genelex is the first firm in the world to offer genetic drug reaction testing directly to the public." What I like about Genelex is that they also offer DNA testing for nutritional genetics, drug reactions, ancestry, and identity.

DNA traditionally had been used to identify people, mostly in forensic or paternity or relationship cases. Then a few years ago, companies began to test DNA for ancestry, which appeals also to genealogists, family historians, and oral historians.

The use of DNA outside of court rooms and forensic laboratories and outside of government and university databases brought DNA to consumers of health care as well as to genealogists interested in molecular genealogy. University laboratories and archaeology research institutes began using the science of archaeogenetics.

Anthropologists who looked at HLA markers, those leukocytes or white blood cells and physicians or scientists who were interested in tissue typing for blood, marrow, and organ transplant donors worked with DNA to identify similar matches, people whose tissues and blood or marrow typing matched close enough for a transplant to take.

You had scientists who studied ancient DNA from fossils and mummies expand the science of archaeogenetics and population geneticists studying migrations of ancient peoples and the routes they took. When ancient and present day comparisons of genetic markers left trails that matched with archaeological relics, new branches of molecular genetics grew.

The science is still emerging, using DNA testing in more ways. Now, we have nutrition and genetics and drug testing and genetics. And there's so much more to arrive that will be available to the general consumer of healthcare, ancestry searching, and identity. From being a spectator in life watching new avenues of DNA testing unfold, the consumer now has the chance to become more involved in participating in and learning about how many ways DNA testing can benefit an individual at any age.

When I went back to Genelex's Web site to explore more material on DNA testing for a variety of purposes, I realized, the consumer has more choices than ever before and still more on the horizon. DNA testing is all about nourishment. From nutrigenomics to drug reaction testing, strategies for better health is being covered from all angles. Perhaps you—as a consumer—want a healthier eating guideline customized to your genetic signature. Maybe you'd like a report on how your genes (and body) respond to certain chemicals, medicines, or substances. Whether it's a prescription drug or specific medicines or supplements that you buy over the counter, several genes are tested to see how your body metabolizes the substance. Not every gene in your body is tested to see how they respond to food or medicine—just specific genes and markers.

The science is new and changing, but the future is attractive to general consumers. You don't need a science background to begin your research on how your own body responds to what you put into it and what comes it from the environment.

To begin, consumers need to become more involved in learning about what scientists and physicians are researching and why, and how all these new findings apply to you. To become more involved as a consumer means being able to access information that evaluates the research, that finds credibility or flaws, and that helps you take more responsibility in your own maintenance.

That's why I believe DNA testing can open doors. Even with guarded caution, the benefits are to be explored and discussed. If you have already had your DNA tested for ancestry or identity, consider these new ways in which DNA testing can help you draw up a plan for eating and for any way you take care of your body— from exercise planning and nutrition to medicines and supplements if and when you need them, to making lifestyle changes for better health.

Consumers can learn a lot from news releases, including learning to understand where to begin to educate themselves about their genes. Some of these releases come from universities engaged in research, some from laboratories and genetic testing companies, some from the government, and from other scientific sources. Professionals in molecular genetics and in healthcare need to understand that an open door policy for public education, teaching oneself about DNA is good. To become more informed leads to becoming more involved in consumer's groups for understanding what "gene hunters" are doing.

Science has become so technical that most scientific journal articles are not understood by most consumers without science training. There has to be a midway point. So far, it's the media that translates scientific terminology into plain language for the consumer. Going one step farther, the medical journalist translates the scientific journals into articles and books whereby people with no science background can learn about their genes.

Finally, learning about how one's genes respond to food or drugs is another rung up on the ladder of self-education about how your body works. That's why there's the mass media for the consumer, the popular medical magazines that bring the consumer closer to healthcare professionals, and finally, the scientific and medical journal articles discussing the research. At the top are the evaluators who let the consumers know which research studies were flawed, and that usually filters down through the mass media.

What some scientists call 'snake oil' may either be harmful or may be a forgotten remedy based on plants that worked. For example, honey, cinnamon, and sesame oil. All three will resist bacteria and in the ancient past were used on minor wounds. A century ago colloidal silver was used on scratches to keep out bacteria.

In the Civil War days, it was used on wounds. Today, you can still make your own, inexpensively, but be careful buying brands containing aluminum. In the dentist's chair, colloidal silver mouthwash works as well as some of the more recent remedies such as washing your mouth with harsh substances that can cause ulcers in the mouth. The point is to check out the mechanisms that review accuracy in whatever you read. If you go the homeopathic or naturopathic route, make sure what you use does no harm for your individual genetic response. How do you metabolize what goes into your body? Genetic testing can help here.

When it comes to genetic testing, you can learn a lot from news releases— at least as a starting point in your research and education about your genes. Bioscience communicators have a role to play as interpreters between consumer and scientist. When I took my master's degree in English with a writing emphasis, it was through a graduate scholarship award in science writing. In genetics, being the communicator means bridging the gap between the growing body of knowledge in science and the consumer who might not even know what DNA is. If you have no science knowledge, start by reading press releases to open the first set of doors to understanding more about your genes, markers, and DNA.

What Consumers Can Learn From News Releases

NIGMS Awards $35 Million to UCSD-Led Consortium to Map Metabolic Pathways in Cells

According to a UCSD media release of August 11, 2003, the University of California, San Diego (UCSD) will lead an ambitious national effort to produce a detailed understanding of the structure and function of lipids—cellular fats and oils implicated in a wide range of diseases, including heart disease, stroke, cancer, diabetes and Alzheimer's disease.

The five-year, $35 million grant from the National Institute of General Medical Sciences (NIGMS) will support more than 30 researchers at 18 universities, medical research institutes, and companies across the United States, who will work together in a detailed analysis of the structure and function of lipids. The principal investigator of this collaboration is Edward Dennis, PhD, professor of chemistry and biochemistry in UCSD's Division of Physical Sciences and UCSD's School of Medicine.

Dennis notes that while sequencing the human genome was a scientific landmark, it is just the first step in understanding the diverse array of systems and processes within and among cells. Establishment of this consortium is a significant step in an emerging field called "metabolomics," or the study of metabolites, chemical compounds that "turn on or off cellular responses to food, friend, or foe," he explained.

Lipids are a water-insoluble subset of metabolites central to the regulation and control of normal cellular function, and to disease. Stored as an energy reserve for the cell, lipids are vital components of the cell membrane, and are involved in communication within and between cells. For example, one class of lipids, the sterols, includes estrogen and testosterone.

The initial phases of the project, known as Lipid Metabolites and Pathways Strategy (LIPID MAPS), will be aimed at characterizing all of the lipid metabolites in one type of cell. The term "Lipidomics" is used to describe the study of lipids and their complex changes and interactions within cells. Because this task is too extensive for a single laboratory to complete, researchers at participating centers will each focus on isolating and characterizing all of the lipids in a single class.

This information will then be combined into a database at <http://www.lipidmaps.org> to identify networks of interactions amongst lipid metabolites and to make this information available to other researchers. Shankar Subramaniam, Ph.D., professor of chemistry and bioengineering at UCSD's Jacobs School of Engineering and San Diego Supercomputer Center, will coordinate this aspect of the project.

The cell type selected for study is the macrophage, best known for its role in immune reactions, for example scavenging bacteria and other invaders in the body. Macrophage cells from mice will be used, rather than human cells, because a "library" of mouse cells exists with specific genetic mutations. By studying cells missing certain genes, the research team will attempt to identify what genes code for those enzymes key in synthesis and processing of lipid metabolites. Christopher Glass, M.D., Ph.D., professor of cellular and molecular medicine at UCSD's School of Medicine, will coordinate the macrophage biology and genomics aspects of the consortium.

According to Dennis, one of the most difficult aspects of this project will be to ensure that all the participating research sites are using identical methods. "There has never been an effort to detect all the lipid metabolites in a cell and to quantify the amounts of these lipids," says Dennis. "In order to be able take the data gathered by each lab and put them together to develop new ideas about interactions between lipid metabolites, it is essential to develop new technologies and methods and to standardize them so that they can be applied in the same way at each research site."

Once the researchers have developed these methods and used them to identify and quantify the lipid metabolites in the mouse macrophage, the methods can be applied to gather other information about lipid metabolites in cells. The researchers plan to study the time and dose-dependent effects of lipopolysaccharide, or LPS, a component of the cell walls of many bacteria, on macrophages.

Dennis' lab has studied the effects of LPS on macrophages for the last 20 years. A world authority on these effects, Dennis says that this large-scale, cross-institutional collaboration will create an understanding of LPS' effects on lipid metabolism in unprecedented detail, and set the stage for examining other macrophage effectors such as oxidized LDL, the so-called bad cholesterol which leads to atherosclerosis.

A detailed understanding of lipid metabolism will be valuable in drug design. Most people are already familiar with one class of drugs that interfere with lipid metabolism: the non-steroidal anti-inflammatory drugs (NSAIDs), which include aspirin and ibuprofen. These drugs block the synthesis of prostaglandins, a large group of chemicals secreted by macrophages that causes pain, inflammation and an immunological response.

Statins, which a large number of Americans take daily to lower their cholesterol levels, also dramatically alter lipid metabolites. With a detailed knowledge of each step in the lipid metabolic pathways, more effective drugs with fewer side effects can be designed to combat heart disease and a plethora of other diseases of lipid metabolism.

In addition to UCSD, participants in the LIPID MAPS consortium are: Avanti Polar Lipids, Inc.; Duke University Medical School; Georgia Institute of Technology; University of California, Irvine; University of Colorado School of Medicine; University of Texas Southwestern Medical School; and Vanderbilt University Medical School. Additional collaborators will include scientists from Applied Biosystems; Boston University School of Medicine; Harvard Medical School; Medical College of Georgia; Medical University of South Carolina; National Jewish Medical and Research Center; Scripps Research Institute; University of Michigan Medical School; University of Utah; and Virginia Commonwealth University. For more information on the grant program, see the related release at http://www.nigms.nih.gov/news/releases/ .

DNA testing isn't only for anthropologists. It includes but goes beyond forensic research in identity. It expands from population genetics to cellular nourishment. It's for the general consumer with no science training, the physician, the genetics counselor, and the nutritionist. DNA testing is for the genealogist and the oral historian. And there are many more applications of DNA testing/genetic testing on the horizon.

According to Genelex's Web site (copyright 2003) at: http://www.healthanddna.com/pharmacogenetics.html, (reprinted here with permission):

"The relatively new and emerging fields of pharmacogenetics and pharmacogenomics study how differences in individual genetic makeup affect the processing of drugs. Pharmacogenetics largely focuses on specific genes, such as drug-metabolizing enzymes, while pharmacogenomics deals with the entire human genome, including genes for numerous proteins in the body, such as transporters, receptors, and the entire signaling networks that respond to drugs and move them through the system.

We have known for about a half-century that individuals respond to the same drug and dosage in very different ways because of genetic variations called polymorphisms. The first studies of what came to be pharmacogenetics were conducted in the early 1950s and examined drug metabolizing enzyme variants such as those in the Cytochrome P450 family. Research shows that of all the clinical factors such as age, sex, weight, general health and liver function that alter a patient's response to drugs; genetic factors are the most important.

Although the genomes of individuals are 99.9% identical, the 0.1% difference means we have as many as 3 million polymorphisms, the most common being the single nucleotide polymorphism (SNP). Detecting polymorphisms is the foundation of pharmacogenetics.

Misdosing of drugs in America costs more than $100 billion dollars a year, and is a leading cause of death. Pharmacogenetics helps to explain why some individuals respond to drugs and others don't. It can also help doctors identify individuals needing higher or lower doses and who will respond to a drug thera-peutically and who might have an adverse drug reaction.

Currently, the clinical use of pharmacogenetics is limited, with the most extensive use in Scandinavia to treat psychiatric illnesses. The technology is, how-ever, steadily moving into other geographic and medical areas, especially cardiol-ogy and cancer treatment.

The Human Genome Project has been an incredible boon to pharmacoge-nomics. As new data are decoded and more precise maps produced, we can begin to understand what specific genes are and how they function. We can also better appreciate the significance of DNA variation among individuals. Preventative medicine and pharmacogentics are the first disciplines to benefit from this vastly increased understanding of human diversity.

Better understanding of the variation in the enzymes involved in drug metab-olism and in the drug targets themselves will help explain why there is so much variation in drug response. We are now able to test for these variations before pre-scribing, and reduce the amount of human experimentation (and associated health care costs) needed to find the best therapy or dose. Drug companies can now develop drugs which are designed by choice, rather than happenstance, to be effective in wide range of the population.

Predictive genetics is revolutionizing health care. DNA tests and personalized drug therapies are shifting the medical paradigm from detection and treatment to prediction and prevention and vastly increasing the efficacy, safety, and variety of therapeutic drugs. Predictive tests and preventative therapies reduce costs associ-ated with hospitalization and lost productivity and will lead to a major redistrib-ution of value in the health care industry."

The following material below is reprinted here with permission, copyright Genelex 2003, according to the **Genelex** Web site, at: http://www.healthanddna.com/ drugreactiontest.html.

Drug Reaction Testing

Do not alter the dosage amount or schedule of any drug you are tak-ing without first consulting your doctor or pharmacists.

"Research shows that of all the clinical factors such as age, sex, weight, gen-eral health and liver function that alter a patient's response to drugs, genetic fac-tors are the most important. This information becomes even more crucial when you consider the fact that adverse reactions to prescription drugs are killing about 106,000 Americans each year—roughly three times as many as are killed by automobiles. This makes prescription drugs the fourth leading killer in the U.S., after heart disease, cancer, and stroke.

"We currently offer CYP2D6, CYP2C9, and CYP2C19 screens that can help your physician or druggist predict your particular response to more than a quarter of all prescription drugs. These include such important medications as Coumadin (Warfarin), Prozac, Zoloft, Paxil, Effexor, Hydrocodone, Amitriptyline, Claritin, Cyclobenzaprine, Haldol, Metoprolol, Rythmol, Tagamet, Tamoxifen, Valium, Carisoprodol, Diazepam, Dilantin, Premarin, and Prevacid (and the over-the-counter drugs, Allegra, Dytuss and Tusstat). Click here to view a more complete list of drugs processed through these pathways.

"Approximately half of all Americans have genetic defects that affect how they process these drugs. There are four different types of metabolizers, and we all fall into one of these categories for the variable pathways in Cytochrome P450 (this Cytochrome is responsible for creating the enzymes that process chemicals of all kinds through our bodies.) The easiest way to understand this is to picture a two lane highway.

If you are the first type which is the norm, you would be an EXTENSIVE metabolizer. Both lanes of the highway are open and moving. Medications prescribed in normal doses will be metabolized by your body.

If you are the second type, you would be an INTERMEDIATE metabolizer. This means that one lane of that highway is open and moving and the other lane is not, causing you to metabolize the medications more slowly. In this case you will need a lower dosage, and there is a chance of medications building up in your system causing adverse effects. It is especially important to monitor medications if you are in this category.

"Intermediate metabolizers through the 2C9 pathway, for instance, have an increased risk of bleeding incidences when taking the common blood thinner Coumadin or Warfarin. For this reason, a recent article in the Journal of the American Medical Association, titled *"Association Between CYP2C9 Genetic Variants and Anticoagulation-Related Outcomes During Wayfarin Therapy,"* JAMA, April 3, 2002—Vol. 287, No. 13, recommends screening for CYP2C9 variants to reduce the risk of adverse drug reactions in these patients.

The third type is a POOR metabolizer. In this case both lanes of the highway would be stopped. There is a possiblility that alternate routes can be found, but this type of metabolizer is potentially very dangerous, as there is a great chance for the medication to build up in your system making you very sick, or even killing you. For example, a poor metabolizer of Phenytoin, a common antiepileptic would not be able to process the drug and would actually have an increased rather than decreased risk of seizure if prescribed this drug.

The fourth type of metabolizer is ULTRA EXTENSIVE. This means you have additional lanes for processing, picture an Indy 500 speedway. In this instance, you literally burn through medications. If you were an Ultra extensive metabolizer through the 2D6 pathway and while in surgery and your doctor gave you codeine as a pain killer, you would receive no pain relief because the codeine would be metabolized so fast that it would have little or no effect on you."

The Testing Process

"The process is simple. We send you a blood collection kit in the mail. You can either make an appointment with your doctor or we will provide you with the contact information for a phlebotomist in your area. Blood samples are overnighted to our laboratory and results are typically available in 15 business days.

Currently Available Tests

"**CYP2D6** (cytochrome P450 2D6) is the best studied of the DMEs and acts on one-fourth of all prescription drugs, including the selective serotonin reuptake inhibitors (SSRI), tricylic antidepressants (TCA), betablockers such as Inderal and the Type 1A antiarrhythmics. Approximately 10% of the population has a slow acting form of this enzyme and 7% a super-fast acting form. Thirty-five percent are carriers of a non-functional 2D6 allele, especially elevating the risk of ADRs when these individuals are taking multiple drugs.

Drugs that CYP2D6 metabolizes include Prozac, Zoloft, Paxil, Effexor, Hydrocodone, Amitriptyline, Claritin, Cyclobenzaprine, Haldol, Metoprolol, Rythmol, Tagamet, Tamoxifen, and the over-the-counter diphenylhydramine drugs, Allegra, Dytuss, and Tusstat. CYP2D6 is responsible for activating the pro-drug codeine into its active form and the drug is therefore inactive in CYP2D6 slow metabolizers.

CYP2C9 (cytochrome P450 2C9) is the primary route of metabolism for Coumadin (Warfarin). Approximately 10% of the population are carriers of at least one allele for the slow-metabolizing form of CYP2C9 and may be treatable with 50% of the dose at which normal metabolizers are treated. Other drugs metabolized by CYP2C9 include Amaryl, Isoniazid, Sulfa, Ibuprofen, Amitriptyline, Dilantin, Hyzaar, THC (tetrahydrocannabinol), Naproxen, and Viagra.

CYP2C19 (cytochrome P450 2C19) is associated with the metabolism of Carisoprodol, Diazepam, Dilantin, Premarin, and Prevacid.

Other tests in the planning stage at the time this book went to press include:

NAT2 (N-acetyltransferase 2) is a second-step DME that acts on Isoniazid, Procainamide, and Azulfidine. The frequency of the NAT2 "slow acetylator" in various worldwide populations ranges from 10% to more than 90%.

"The advantages of Genelex's consumer genetic testing include:

Safety. Decrease the chance that you will be the victim of an adverse drug reaction. More than 100,000 hospitalized Americans die of adverse drug reactions and two million outpatients have serious episodes each year. Knowledge of your DNA Drug Reaction Profile may help your physician or druggist prevent this from happening.

Efficacy. Prescription drugs on the market today are usually prescribed by trial and error because they have been tested and approved in a "one size fits all" fashion. If you eliminate a particular drug more rapidly than the norm, taking the normal dose may be a complete waste of time. The drug simply will not work as prescribed, and it may take a while to discover this.

Responsibility. Play a more active role in your health, your family's health, and in healthcare at large. DNA testing for drug reactions is just coming onto the market and you, the consumer, can help all of us take this major step toward better medicine."

"Check out the common drugs processed by enzymes that Genelex tests. Genelex currently offers "DNA Prescription Drug Reaction Profiles that test 2D6,2C9, and 2c19 functionality. The table below lists many commonly prescribed drugs that are metabolized through these pathways in the Cytochrome P-450 system. If your medication is not on the list, ask your pharmacist or physician about the metabolic pathway."

Common drugs prescribed by physicians or bought over-the-counter are processed by enzymes. Look at Genelex's Drug List by clicking on the PDF file to see Genelex's Drug list. See below, reprinted with permission, copyright Genelex, 2003. Or go to their Web site at: http://www.healthanddna.com/drugreactiontest.html and click on the PDF file to view the list of drugs at: http://www.healthanddna.com/drugchart.PDF. What you're looking for is prescription drug reaction testing.

Your body metabolizes drugs differently than another person based on your individual genetic response. So look at the drug metabolization guide. Is your prescription drug listed there? What about drugs or supplements you buy over the counter? The typeset formatting is different on the PDF file. So look at the list below at: http://www.healthanddna.com/drugchart.PDF.

On the PDF file, you'll note that the formatting for numbers such as 2D6 is different in the PDF file than reprinted here due to formatting differences between a paperback book and the PDF file on the Web. So to get the correct formatting of the numbers such as 2D6 lined up with the correct drugs, use the PDF file to do your looking rather than the book, which is just a list of drugs tested. The PDF file has the correct numbers lined up with the correct names of the drugs.

Below is just a list of the drugs to give you an idea of what drug reaction test-ing is about and the names of the drugs listed. So use Genelex's PDF file, not the book if you want to see what numbers are lined up with what drugs. Below is to give you an idea of how a drug metabolization guide may be of benefit to a con-sumer when talking to your physician. The point is for you to learn how to become more involved in researching how your genes respond to what you put in your body.

Drug List

Prescription Drug Reaction Testing
Drug Metabolization Guide
(Reprinted here with permission, copyright Genelex 2003.)

Substrates Metabolized through Cytochrome P-450

2D6
acetaminophen citalopram galanthamine norfluoxetine saquinavir
ajmaline clomipramine gallopamil nortriptyline sertinodole
alprenolol clozapine guanoxan octopamine setraline
amiflamine cobenzoline halofantrine olanzapine sildenafil
aminopyrine codeine haloperidol omeprazole S-metoprolol
amiodarone debrisoquine ibogaine ondansetron sparteine
amitriptyline delavirdine iloperidone opipramol tamoxifen
amphetamine deprenyl imipramine orto=Phebylphenol tamsulosin
amprenavir desipramine indinavir oxedrine tauromustine
aprinidine desmethylcitalopramindoramin oxycodone terfenadine
astemizole dexfenfluramine lidocaine parathion terguride
azelastine dextromethorphan lisuride paroxetine theophylline
benzydamine dextrromethorphan loratidine perhexiline thioridazine
bepranolol diazonin maprotline perphenazine timolol
bisoprolol diclofenac mequitazine phenacetin tolterodine
brofaramine diethyldithocarbamate methyl ester
methadone phenformin tramadol bromoperidol dihydrocodeine
methlyamphetamine pranidipine trifluperidol
buflomedil diltiazem methoxyamphetamine pregnenolone trimipramine
bufuralol diprafenone methoxyphenamine procainamide tropisetron
bunitrolol dolasetron metoprolol progesterone tryptamine
bupivacaine donepezil mexiletine promethazine tyramine
buthylamphetamine doxepin mianserin propafenone venlafaxine

captopril encainide milameline propranolol zolpidem
carteolol estradiol milameline propylajamaline zotepine
carvedilol estradiol minaprine prprofol zuclopenthixol
chlorophyros ethylmorphine mirtazapine quanoxan
chloropromazine ezlopitant nelfinavir mesylate quetiapine
chlorpheniramine flecainide nevirapine ranitidine
chlorzoxazone flunarizine nicardipine remoxipride
cilostazol fluoxetine nicotine retinol
cinnarizine fluperlapine nifedipine risperidone
fluphenazine norcodeine ritonavir
fluvastatin ropivacaine
fluvoxamine

Substrates Metabolized through Cytochrome P-450
2C19 2C9 ctd' 2C9 ctd'
amitriptyline aceclofenac tropisetron
citalopram acenocoumarol valproic acid
clominpramine acetaminophen venlafaxine
cyclophosphamide
alosetron verapamil
diazepam aminopyrine warfarin
imipramine amitriptyline zafirlukast
lansoprazole amitriptyline zidovudine
nelfinavir amprenavir zileuton
omeprazole antipyrine zolpidem
pantoprozole arachidonic acid
phenytoin artelinic acid
rabeprazole benzopyrene
bufuralol
butadiene monoxide
candesartan
carvedilol
celecoxib
chlorpyrifos
cinnarizine
cisapride
cloazapine
cyclophosphamide
dapsone
deprenyl

desmethyladinazolam
desogestrel
dextromethorphan
diallyl disulfide
diazepam
dibenzoanthracene
dibenzylfluorescein

**Inhibitors Metabolized through
Cytochrome P-450
2C19 2C9 2D6**
cimetidine amiodarone amiodarone
flebamate fluconazole celecoxib
fluoxetine fluvastatin chlorpheniramine
fluvoxamine fluvoxamine cimetidine
ketoconazole
isoniazid clomipramine
lansoprazole lovastatin cocaine
omeprazole paroxetine doxorubicin?
paroxetine phenylbutazone fluoxetine
ticlopidine probenicid? halofantrine
sertraline levomepromazine
sulfaphenazole methadone
teniposide mibefradil
trimethoprim moclobemide
zafirlukast paroxetine
quinidine
ranitidine
red-haloperidol
ritonavir
terbinafine
chlorpheniramine
cimetidine
clomipramine
cocaine
doxorubicin?
fluoxetine
halofantrine
levomepromazine
methadone

mibefradil
moclobemide
paroxetine
quinidine
ranitidine
red-haloperidol
ritonavir
terbinafine

Inducers Metabolized through Cytochrome P-450
2C9 2C19 2D6
rifampin carbamazepine dexamethasone
secobarbital norethindrone rifampin?
rifampin

For immediate consultation Call 800-TEST-DNA (800–837–8362)
Hours 7:00 AM to 6:00 PM PST, 10:00 AM to 9:00 PM EST, fax 206–219–4000,
3000 First Avenue, Suite One, Seattle, WA 98121
E-mail: info@genelex.com Web: www.genelex.com
Se habla español. ©2003 Genelex Corporation

Scientists and Physicians Comment on Pharmacogenetics

Question: Where would consumers (with no science background) begin to search and learn about pharmacogenetics?

——Original Message——
From: Prakash Nadkarni
To: Anne Hart
Sent: Friday, August 15, 2003 9:19 AM
Subject: RE: query by writer

Hi Anne,

The world's biggest library, of course, is the Web (if you use a good tool like Google), and of course, you can walk to your nearest medical school if you need technical information—I know they shouldn't prevent use you from using the reference section unless they happen to be total A-holes (some of the Ivy league libraries are like that).

Re: interviews—E-mail is not a good medium for "interviews", though instant messaging probably is (I'm not sure how many scientists use it, though—I avoid it myself because I don't like to be interrupted while I'm in the middle of something.)

How it's going to help the average consumer—I don't know. My attitude is guarded optimism.

The cost of developing a new drug is frightfully high. If a new drug turns out to have an adverse effect that might result in its being pulled from the market, then, **if** it could be shown that this adverse effect has a clear-cut pharmacogenetic basis AND there is a very simple test that could detect susceptibility, then the drug could still be on the market.

- The flip side here: the really scary adverse effects are not all that common, they may occur in 1 of a 1000 individuals or less. Then you require a very large number of subjects to PROVE a pharmacogenetic basis for that adverse event. This costs a lot of money, and the FDA may not wait that long to pull the drug from the market if safer alternatives already exist.

(There may be gray areas, though—troglitazone was one of the first of a new family of antidiabetic agents—the thiazolidinediones, or PPAR-gamma activators—that work by a unique mechanism. It was pulled from the market because of liver toxicity, but when this happened, many patients whose lives had been dramatically improved by the drug actually complained to the FDA that they were perfectly happy to continue taking it.

Fortunately, newer and safer drugs from the same chemical family were developed, such as rosiglitazone and pioglitazone. However, we don't know as yet whether there is a clearly and easily characterizable pharmacogenetic mechanism for thiazolidinediones-induced liver toxicity, so I'm really citing this as an example of a valuable drug that deserves and could get a second chance.

Similarly, if a genetic test indicates that a particular individual is potentially vulnerable to a dangerous adverse effect (for a potentially life-saving drug (e.g. an anticancer agent) which has dangerous side effects), then one could avoid this drug and seek an alternative drug to treat the same condition.

Re: Pharmacogenetics and diet, the lactose-intolerance of Han Chinese (as well as their greatly increased susceptibility to alcohol hangover with much more modest quantities of liquor) is well known, as is the fact that African-Americans require a larger quantity of eye drops to dilate the pupil prior to a retinal exam compared to people with light-colored eyes.

The complications here—it's not just a single gene for susceptibility, it's multiple genes (not to mention interaction of genes with environmental factors) that makes research in the field so damned difficult. Even when you have two people with the same susceptibility gene, the response to the same drug may vary ten-fold,—there are numerous other genes that we haven't considered in the study that are responsible for the variation.

Genes and environment—repeated exposure to certain environmental agents may induce the expression of genes that result in greater tolerance to the agent. The ability of Russians to tolerate an astonishing amount of vodka (that they've been consuming since very young) is a case in point.

Also genes and age: study after study has shown that people who are susceptible to substance abuse (tobacco, booze etc.) are much more likely to get hooked if they're exposed to the substance during or before adolescence, which is why you have the laws about selling this stuff to minors. (We haven't studied brain plasticity enough—we don't know what's magical about the adolescence cut-off, but we do know that people who learn a foreign language by being immersed in that culture can learn speak it without an accent if exposed before adolescence, but not after.)

Hope this helps, and good luck with your book.

Regards,
Prakash
——
Prakash Nadkarni, MD
Associate Professor
Yale Center for Medical Informatics
New Haven, CT

To: 'Anne Hart'
Sent: Friday, August 15, 2003 12:07 PM
Subject: Re: query by journalist

Dear Ms. Hart:

Thank you for contacting the National Institute of General Medical Sciences, a component of the National Institutes of Health. NIGMS supports research in pharmacology, and more specifically, in pharmacogenetics. I know that you also contacted Dr. Rochelle Long at NIGMS, so I am responding on her behalf as well. NIGMS supports a network of pharmacogenetic researchers, listed at the following URL: http://www.nigms.nih.gov/pharmacogenetics/research_network.html. You could take a look at their research project summaries to get a sense for the kind of research that is going on. Also, you could try a Google News search on pharmacogenetics and/or pharmacogenomics to find published interviews/stories for context for your book.

Regarding consumer information, NIGMS has published two educational brochures on the topic. Online versions are posted at:
http://www.nigms.nih.gov/funding/medforyou.html

and
http://www.nigms.nih.gov/news/science_ed/genepop/

If you would like hard copies of either or both of these borchures, send an email request to pub_info@nigms.nih.gov.

Regarding the availability of genetic tests:

There are at least 2 pharmacogenetics tests that are widely available and offered by certified commercial clinical testing laboratories: TPMT and CYP2D6. There is no current standard for the widespread use of pharmacogenetics testing—yet. It is performed either as a difficult case referral to a tertiary care setting (e.g. Mayo Clinic), or due to patient interest in seeking it out (e.g. based on a web advertisement).

Physicians are divided on when adverse side effects that occur in rare patients should be dealt with: after they occur, or anticipated and prevented. Sometimes these events are uncomfortable (e.g. lack of pain control after taking codeine; once caught, a morphine based drug like vicodin can be used instead); sometimes these events are life-threatening (e.g. myelosuppression after an anticancer drug; once recognized, a lesser dose of the agent can be used).

The most modern research scientific approach is to tailor the drug choice and drug dose to the patient up front. But there are instances where this just simply isn't the prevailing standard of care, either for economic reasons, or for reasons of time, or for valid reasons (e.g. PTT testing in hospital after warfarin is performed, rather than pre-prescriptive genotyping makes sense, since genotype isn't the only influence on clotting time; diet matters too).

If you are interested in researching the industry angle:

Meeting report from last year's meeting of the NIH Pharmacogenetics Research Network (see especially the second keynote by Rebecca Eisenberg):
http://www.nigms.nih.gov/pharmacogenetics/2002meeting_report.html

Members of the NIH Pharmacogenetics Research Network Industry Liaison Group:
http://www.nigms.nih.gov/pharmacogenetics/PRN_industry_liaison_roster.html

These folks, from small and big pharma and biotech, may be able to give you the view from the trenches.

A publication called The Scientist published a relatively savvy article on the topic last year; find the story at: http://www.the-scientist.com/yr2002/sep/research1_020930.html

(you have to register but it's free access to the full text)

I hope some of this information is helpful to you.

Alison Davis
Office of Communications and Public Liaison
NIGMS. NIH

——Original Message——
From: "Esteban Gonzalez Burchard, M.D."
To: "Anne Hart"
Sent: Thursday, August 14, 2003 9:33 PM
Subject: Re: Pharmacogenetics: What Can You Comment About Regarding Pharmacogenetics for the General Consumer?

Hi Anne:

I have attached a section that I wrote as part of a grant. You can use this as you please. As of today, there are not that many examples that are of use to the public. However there are examples developed at St. Jude Children's Hospital in Memphis in which they can test for mutations in the
drug metabolizing enzyme that metabolizes specific chemotherapy drugs. In doing so, physicians can now identify who will be at risk for toxic levels of the chemotherapy drug.

The best publicly known example is alcohol and facial flushing in Asians. This is due to a genetic variant in the Alcohol Dehydrogenase Enzyme. This is a perfect example of a pharmacogenetic response.

Esteban

****

It is well established that among U.S. residents of similar socioeconomic status, there is greater cardiovascular morbidity and mortality among African Americans and Latino Americans than among Caucasians.[1–4] In addition, there is marked clinical heterogeneity in the prevalence and
treatment of hypertension among specific ethnic and racial groups.

Specifically, there are marked differences in drug response to antihypertensive therapy with angiotensin converting enzyme inhibitors (ACE-I) among African Americans than among Caucasians.[5,6]. Although there are many potential explanations for this observation, including
environmental and socioeconomic factors, one potential explanation is that the genetic predisposition to hypertension and to differences in drug response differs among racial and ethnic groups. In particular, we propose that genetic differences may explain, in part, the differences in response to ACE inhibitors between African American and Caucasian Americans.[7]

Hypertension among U.S. Populations: Cardiovascular disease is a substantial public health problem and a leading cause of death for all U.S. ethnic and racial minorities. The impact of premature morbidity from cardiovascular disease is devastating in terms of personal loss, pain,
suffering, and effects on families and loved ones. The annual national economic impact of cardiovascular disease is estimated at $259 billion as measured in health care expenditures, medications, and lost productivity due to disability and death. <http://raceandhealth.hhs.gov/3rdpgBlue/Cardio/3pgGoalsCardio.htm> A major modifiable risk factor for cardiovascular disease is high blood pressure (hypertension).

Disparities exist in the prevalence of risk factors for cardiovascular disease. Racial and ethnic minorities have higher rates of hypertension, tend to develop hypertension at an earlier age, and are less likely to respond to conventional antihypertensive therapies to control their high blood pressure.[6] For example, from 1988 to 1994, 35 percent of black males ages 20 to 74 had hypertension compared with 25 percent of all men. When age differences are taken into account, Mexican-American men and women also have elevated blood pressure rates. Among adult women, the age-adjusted prevalence of overweight continues to be higher for black women (53 percent) and Mexican-American women (52 percent) than for Caucasian women (34 percent). Although there are multiple potential explanations for the observed differences in the prevalence of hypertension, possible explanation include biologic or genetic differences.

Clinical and racial heterogeneity in response to treatment of hypertension:

Numerous large-scale clinical trials of therapy for heart failure and hypertension over the past decade have shown improvements in outcome with angiotensin converting enzyme inhibitors (ACE-I).[8–13] Interestingly, data from the second Vasodilator-Heart Failure Trial (V-HeFT II) indicated that although enalapril therapy was associated with significant reduction in the
risk of death from any cause among white patients, no such benefit was observed among black patients.[14] In addition, the Beta-Blocker Evaluation of Survival Trail found significant benefits with the beta blocker bucindolol among white patients but not black patients.[15] A reduced
response to ACE inhibitors in black patients as compared to white patients is well documented.

Decreases in blood pressure in black patients with hypertension have been shown to be less than white patients given similar doses of ACE inhibitors [16] and beta blockers.[17] Taken together, these data may suggest that there are racial/ethnic differences in therapeutic response to the treatment of heart failure and hypertension among different racial/ethnic groups. More importantly, these trials have raised the possibility that black patients with heart failure and hypertension may not benefit from commonly used doses of recommended therapies to the same extent as white patients.

Genetic differences among races: Naturally occurring genetic variants or polymorphisms of genes are an important source of genetic diversity. Single nucleotide polymorphisms (SNPs) account for over 90% of all human DNA polymorphism.[18] It is well established that there are differences in allele frequencies among various ethnic groups.[19,20] By determining the degree of disease risk associated with particular alleles, in conjunction with the allele frequency for a defined population, one can derive information about the population attributable risk, which is relevant to the public health impact for that population.

Genetics of Hypertension: In favor of genetic factors being an important in the pathogenesis and treatment of hypertension are observations from studies in families, twins, and clinical pharmacologic trials performed in ethnically diverse groups.[6,21–28] Although there have been no systematic genome-wide screens performed across racial or ethnic populations, there have been individual investigations in African Americans, Mexican Americans, Chinese and Caucasians.[29–33] All of these investigations found linkage between loci and hypertension. Interestingly, most of these loci differed by the ethnic population studied, suggesting genetic heterogeneity. This may suggest that there are "ethnic specific" genetic risk factors that are associated with hypertension in different racial and/or ethnic groups with resulting differences in drug response to antihypertensive drugs.

Genetic sequence variants among hypertension candidate genes: There is increasing evidence to suggest that drug metabolism alone does not account for the observed interindividual variability in drug disposition or response, but that other processes, including drug transport, are important determinants of drug disposition.[34,35] Drug transporters in the gastrointestinal tract are a major determinant of oral bioavailability of drugs whereas transporters in the kidney and liver are major determinants of renal and hepatic clearances.

Transporters in specific tissues (e.g., the blood brain barrier) control tissue specific distribution of drugs. The pharmacokinetics of the ACE inhibitors have been reviewed recently.[36,37] It is important to note that the absorption of several ACE inhibitors is low (approximately 40% of an oral dose is absorbed) and variable and appears to be controlled by the oligopeptide transporter, Pept1.[38]

Several ACE inhibitors are eliminated by active secretion in the kidney, and appear to interact with renal organic anion transporters (e.g., OAT1 and OAT3). Thus, genetic variation in transporters involved in absorption and elimination of ACE inhibitors will contribute to variation in drug response. It is possible that variants of these transporters present in different frequencies among various ethnic populations may explain (in part) ethnic differences in response to ACE inhibitors.

Summary and Significance: Currently available data indicate that cardiovascular morbidity and mortality disproportionately affect U.S. ethnic and racial minority groups. This proposal is the first phase of a systematic effort to identify biologic and genetic explanations for these differences in drug response to conventional antihypertensive therapies. We will recruit a local cohort of ethnically diverse subjects who will undergo phenotype analysis and genetic testing of candidate genes thought to be involved in the transport of anithypertensive drugs.

As part of the overall PMT project these genetic variants will be further tested with in vitro functional assays to determine the biologic relevancy of the identified genetic variants. As part of future studies, these subjects will be called back to participate in further pharmacokinetic testing. Subjects will be stratified by their respective genotypes and then undergo pharmacologic testing with conventional antihypertensive therapies.

These investigations will allow us to determine whether pharmacogenetic relationships exist. More importantly, these investigations will allow us to identify ethnic-specific differences in drug response by genotype. The overall aims of this proposal are to better understand the genetic factors that may contribute to the increased disparity from cardiovascular and hypertension morbidity and mortality seen among ethnically diverse populations. These aims are consistent with those established by Healthy People, which are to reduce disparities in health among different population groups.

Esteban González Burchard, M.D.
Pulmonary and Critical Care Medicine
Department of Medicine
University of California, San Francisco

Mailing Address:
  University of California, San Francisco
  Box 0833
  San Francisco, California 94143

Shipping Address:
  UCSF DNA Bank/Lung Biology Center
  San Francisco General Hospital
  Bldg 30, 5th Floor, Room 3501H
  1001 Potrero Avenue
  San Francisco, California 94110

From: Wein, Harrison (NIH/OD)
To: 'Anne Hart'
Sent: Friday, August 15, 2003 11:36 AM
Subject: RE: Thanks for replying

I just got the latest table of contents for *Environmental Health Perspectives*, and noticed that they feature pharmacogenomics in their new issue. There are a couple of articles in the issue. Here's the link: http://ehp.niehs.nih.gov/txg/docs/2003/111–11/toc.html.

Harrison

From: "Daniel Rubin"
To: "Anne Hart"
Subject: Re: query by writer
Date: Friday, August 15, 2003 5:15 PM

You can find educational information on our PharmGKB web site that should provide much of what you're looking for:
http://www.pharmgkb.org/do/serve?id=resources.education

Also, NIH as an educational brochure on pharmacogenetics for the public that may give you what you're looking for in terms of how this will benefit the public: http://www.nigms.nih.gov/funding/medforyou.html

I recall that Time magazine did a very nice piece in 2001 on pharmacogenomics directly addressing exactly what you're talking about, and that you should be able to find in a community public library.

Regards,

Daniel

UCSD Scientists Develop Novel Ways to Screen Molecules Using Conventional CDs and Compact Disk Players

Molecules attached to CDs in new techniques can screen for proteins. According to a UCSD August 18, 2003 press release, chemists at the University of California, San Diego have developed a novel method of detecting molecules with a conventional compact disk player that provides scientists with an inexpensive way to screen for molecular interactions and a potentially cheaper alternative to medical diagnostic tests.

A paper detailing their development will appear this week in an advance on-line edition of the journal Organic and Biomolecular Chemistry (http://xlink.rsc.org/?DOI=b306391G) and in the printed journal's September 21st issue.

"Our immediate goal is to use this new technology to solve basic scientific questions in the laboratory," says Michael Burkart, an assistant professor of chemistry and biochemistry at UCSD and a coauthor of the paper. "But our eventual hope is that there will be many other applications. Our intention is to make this new development as widely available as possible and to see where others take the technology."

"The CD is by far the most common media format in our society on which to store and read information," says La Clair. "It's portable, you can drop it on the floor and it doesn't break. It's easy to mass produce. And it's inexpensive."

Burkart and James La Clair, a visiting scholar in Burkart's laboratory who initially developed and patented the technique, said that since scientific laboratories often rely on laser light to detect molecules, it made sense to them to design a way to detect molecules using the most ubiquitous laser on the planet—the CD player.

Their technique takes advantage of the tendency for anything adhering to the CD surface to interfere with a laser's ability to read digital data burned onto the CD.

"We developed a method to identify biological interactions using traditional compact disk technology," explains La Clair, who provided the patent rights to the method to UCSD. "Using inkjet printing to attach molecules to the surface of a CD, we identified proteins adhering to these molecules by their interaction with the laser light when read by a CD player."

While usually anything, like a scratch on the CD surface, that would interfere with the detection of the bits of information encoded on a CD would be a drawback, the UCSD researchers actually exploited this error to detect molecules.

"That's the novelty of this," Burkart points out. "We are actually using the error to get our effect."

The typical CD consists of a layer of metal sandwiched between a layer of plastic and a protective lacquer coating. When a CD is burned, a laser creates pits in the metal layer. A CD player uses a laser to translate the series of pits and intervening smooth surface into the corresponding zeros and ones that make up the bits of digital information.

To do molecular screening, the researchers took a CD encoded with digital data, and enhanced the chemical reactivity of the plastic on the readable surface. They then added molecules they wanted to attach to this surface to the empty ink wells of an inkjet printer cartridge and used the printer to "print" the molecules onto the CD. This resulted in a CD with molecules bound to its readable surface in specific locations relative to the pits in the metal layer of the CD encoding the digital information. When the CD with these molecules attached is placed in a CD player, the laser detects a small error in the digital code relative to what is read from the CD without the molecules attached.

To detect proteins or other large molecules in a solution like a blood sample, the modified CD is allowed to react with the sample solution. Like a key that only fits in a certain lock, some proteins bind to specific target molecules. Thus, specific molecules on the surface of a CD can be used to "go fishing" for certain proteins in a sample. The attachment of these proteins will introduce further errors into the reading of the CD. Furthermore, since the molecules on the surface of the CD are at known locations relative to the bits of encoded information, the errors tell the researchers what molecules have attached to their target protein and, thus, whether or not that protein is present in the sample.

"James has even done this using CDs with music, like Beethoven's Fifth Symphony," says Burkart. "And you can actually hear the errors."

"How many people on this planet can actually hear a molecule attached to another molecule?" asks La Clair.

While a few bugs need to be ironed out before the technique can be used to accurately quantify the amount of a given protein in solution, Burkart plans to apply it immediately to help him screen for new compounds in his natural products chemistry research laboratory. Compared to the $100,000 price tag for a fluorescent protein chip reader, he points out, a CD player costs as little as $25.

The researchers envision many other potential applications for this technology outside the laboratory, particularly in the development of inexpensive medical diagnostic tests, now beyond the means of many people around the world, particularly in developing countries.

"In theory, anyone who has a computer with a CD drive could do medical tests in their own home," says La Clair.

The researchers hope that by openly publishing their development in the scientific literature, others will customize the technology in a variety of ways, eventually leading to a wide range of inexpensive new diagnostic kits and other beneficial products.

"We plan to make this fully available and see what people come up with," says Burkart.

For additional information, see: http://discode.ucsd.edu/

Chapter Three

DNA Testing for Nutritional Genomics and Ancestry

What does ancestry have to do with how your genes respond to food or medicine? Certain ethnic groups or 'races' respond in different ways to different medicines, dosages, foods, exercise, illnesses, lifestyle changes, and stress. Since most people have a mixture of genes from several races or ethnic groups going back to prehistoric times, only a DNA test of specific genetic markers or genes can reveal what you're are at risk for regardless of your dominant ethnicity. The genes respond in specific ways to chemicals in the environment and other factors.

That's why you can interpret a report, talk it over with your physician, and tailor what you eat, what drugs you take and the dosages for your condition, to what your genetic expression requires to be healthy. It's looking at you at the cellular level, the molecular level. Most people don't even know what DNA is; or consumers have no science background. So they need an easy to understand consumer's guide to nutritional genomics and pharmacogenetics.

Consumers want to know how their individual, specific genes and possibly their ancestry respond to food—selected foods tailored or prescribed to nourish your individual genetic profile known as your *genetic expression*. Consumer involvement in nutritional genomics is important as it is in pharmacogenetics. How many products need to be tailored to your genes? Food? Medicines? Cosmetics? What else? Let's look at the issues.

Nutritional genomics, often abbreviated as 'nutrigenomics,' is about increasing that success rate. How will science working together with the consumer tackle the issues confronting us as the population ages? Consumer involvement can democratize the science of nutritional genomics by improving diets for better health. You can ask to work on ethics boards or create your own. How is discovering deep ancestry through DNA testing related to the ways that food affects your health?

Ancestry and diet are linked by biology, culture, and choices. It's all about collaborating with your genes. Do you choose your food by habit or biology? Consumers need a guide to DNA testing for nutritional genomics as well as for ancestry and family history. Specific genetic variants *interact* and relate to nutrition.

Learn to interpret the expression of your genes before you count your calories. If you're supposed to eat 'bright' for your 'genotype,' then you begin by mapping your genetic expression and learning how the raw data applies in a practical way to what you consume. This means genetic testing, interpretation, and application to food.

Are you having your DNA tested to see how your genetic signature responds to the medicines you are taking? What's your genetic response to food, medicine, exercise, or nutraceuticals? If you're concerned about adverse reactions, are you having your genes screened, particularly CYP2D6, CYP2C9, and CYP2C19—to see what your particular response is to prescription medicines? What about the food you eat? Can you tailor what you eat to your genotype?

Does Your DNA Have a Core Identity That's Both Cultural and Biological?

Not only can you trace your family history and ancestry with molecular genealogy or gene testing. You can create a DNA and genealogy time capsule. What are the relationships between your deep, ancient ancestry, your DNA, migrations, and how you customize what you eat to your genetic signature or how you tailor any medicine or supplements you take to specific genes and markers?

Are you interested in foods tailored to your genotype and have no science background? How curious are you about pharmacogenetics—exploring how your doctor tailors your medicine to your genes? Thinking about eating bright for your genotype?

What about DNA and Ancestry? Or perhaps you would like to find out the definition of *genomics, proteomics, metabolomics, or lipidomics*? How far can we take familiar genealogy and oral history techniques and link them to DNA testing for a variety of reasons from tailoring what you eat to your DNA to customizing what over-the-counter and prescription drugs your physician wants you to take?

Before you take anything, ask your physician how your genes will respond to what you put into your body. What DNA and other tests can you take that will be responsible, credible, and appropriate measures for your present or future needs?

Genetic Testing When You are Unhappy with Your Doctor's Response to Questions

Back in 1995, as a medical journalist, I felt unhappy with my doctor's response to my questions regarding different treatment methods for the symptoms of menopause. I was in my early fifties then, and before DNA testing was readily available to consumers, I decided to do my own research to find answers to questions.

The commonly prescribed "one-size fits all" estrogen-progestin pills I received from my primary care physician at my HMO as I entered menopause was prescribed with the words, "If you go off your HRT, it would be like a diabetic going off insulin." I didn't quite believe those words, but that's what the doctor said when I asked about when I could go off the HRT. So I took my pills like he said, and within a few months, my cholesterol levels changed for the worse.

The pills worsened my genetic hypertension. Still, the doctor insisted I not stop taking the HRT. I went to another doctor who changed the routine. Instead of taking an estrogen and a progestin pill each day, he prescribed estrogen some days of the month and progestin other days of the month and warned that, "I'd better do something about my hypertension or I'll have to go on 'meds.'" And still, I felt worse on the estrogen and progestin the more months that passed. After eleven months, I dumped the HRT and didn't go back to the HMO. It was time to do some research and become more involved in my own healthcare as a consumer.

At that time, around 1996, all those Web articles on the dark side of soy didn't yet come to my attention. The universities I visited were doing clinical trials with natural soy products for menopause, and magazine articles were telling me I had to have those 29 grams of soy each day for my bones and arteries. I didn't know who to believe. There were magazines warning of too much stimulation to the thyroid from too much soy isoflavones. I didn't know who to believe yet, but what I wanted was information.

Some nurses told me about natural yam-derived progesterone as an alternative to hormone replacement therapy (HRT). At first, not realizing the genetics of hypertension, I thought that the estrogen in HRT was the cause of my dangerously high blood pressure. Using the Internet to access newsgroups and WWW sites, I sought the alternative therapies and tried to find out whether they really worked. Was there anyone out there saying the studies had been flawed? And if so, how could I believe the critic?

What credentials or credibility did he or she have? And if there were no critics saying studies were flawed, perhaps no studies were ever performed? Who was right? So I turned to the medical journals on the shelves at the local Medical School library. I also turned to the Internet and to physicians online willing to answer my questions about these treatments. What I found were people who had the time to answer questions, but none were physicians.

Were there actual physicians online or available willing to answer questions? Who had the time and who had the credibility? Was it true that unproven holistic health and naturopathic or homeopathic remedies that worked a century ago came back now, and did they really work? Was it true that natural ingredients were better, but not used because the big drug companies could make a profit off of them? How much was snake oil and how much was plant-based cures? Who could I believe?

More important, what would work with my body, nasty genetic defects and all? And when my husband needed hernia surgery, how could the Internet answer questions? This was 1995, before genetic testing was available to consumers.

All I had to go by was the awful, scary reactions I had to dental anesthesia when having a compact wisdom tooth removed at age 26. The IV went in, and the next thing I started yelling I can't breathe. What were my genes telling me? Or the carbocaine for the root canal that caused my panic attack, tremors and convulsing, whereas the specific type of mepivacaine with no vasoconstrictors worked well.

And I remained calm without the jitters I usually received from carbocaine that sent my body into a panic response, unleashing catecholamine and other hormones that raise the blood pressure, heart rate, fear, tremors, with slight nausea and convulsing because of the special genetic response to the anesthetic of my more or less defective (or just different) autonomic nervous system. Interestingly, mepivacaine with no vasoconstrictors allowed me to feel calm, centered, and well while having my teeth fixed.

The popular archaeology magazine article clued me in that I might have a defect in my autonomic nervous system by reading a popular archaeology magazine article about ancient Egyptian mummies that mentioned an article in a medical journal. One eye pulled to the corner that shows up on photos or portraits, a withered left side of the face…It was all pointing to my panic disorder. Even an astrologer mentioned Neptune on the rising sign signaling my anxiety gene.

I had inherited this gene from my father, who claimed he was too nervous to ever learn to drive. I never learned to drive either. What I was looking for was more than vague explanations of "anxiety genes." I had to pinpoint the response, that means in my situation, a hyperinsulinism response or insulin resistance, the family's tendency to gain weight in the abdomen and hardly anywhere else, and to explore the possible need for what a decade later became known as "the Syndrome X diet." It all was genetic, or was it? What helped in the beginning of my quest for research was reading the book titled, *The Metabolic Typing Diet* by William Wolcott and Trish Fahey, Broadway Books, NY 2000. This book was an open door to a plan for customizing your diet and preventive medicine.

Of course, back in 1995 and 1996, I couldn't find a DNA test offered to consumers on the Internet. Instead I used the Web to search for alternative medicine and holistic health articles and supplements. Take a look at my article which appeared in **Internet World** 1996 February: 42–44, 46, and 48. The article below is reprinted with permission. It is also mentioned in archives online. See

HEALTHNET NEWS VOL. XI, NO. 4 WINTER 1995, Lyman Maynard Stowe Library University of Connecticut Health Center: http://library.uchc.edu/ departm/hnet/winter95.html

Menopause and Beyond—Alternative Resources and Information Online

Alternative Resources Online for Menopause and Beyond

Through the Internet, you can obtain information your doctor hasn't got time to give you, and talk to people who share your problems.

By Anne Hart

I have found that doctors don't always have the time or breadth of knowledge to discuss alternative, customized solutions to my family's healthcare needs. That's why I turned to the Internet. After searching the Net for Web sites, support groups, or little-known health newsletters, I found dozens of physicians who offered to give me answers to my specific questions via e-mail.

Each member of my family required a different healthcare service and support group to address their particular problems. In my case, I am allergic to synthetic progestin, which eases the side effects of menopause. At the health-maintenance organization (HMO) to which I am a member, I asked my doctor for natural, yam-derived progesterone.

He refused to prescribe it because he said it wasn't yet approved by the FDA, which left me with no alternatives to prevent osteoporosis, for which I'm at high risk. Instead I was put on hormone-replacement therapy, which involves taking oral estrogen. I believed that the oral estrogen was raising my blood pressure sky high. When I mentioned this to my doctor's nurse, she snapped, "Prove it."

So I set off on my journey to prove it. First I checked the **alt.support.menopause** newsgroup, which was extremely helpful. I posted the following question: *Is anyone else using high soy and vegetarian diets, the herb black cohosh, and natural, yam-derived, progesterone cream for menopause—to help prevent bone loss—instead of the usual estrogen and progestin? If so, what are your comments and experiences?*

The replies were practical, useful, and factual, providing medical references, titles of medical journal articles, and book bibliographies, as well as personal experiences and encouragement. For example, one person pointed me to an article entitled "Risks of Estrogens and Progestogens" in the December 1990 issue of *Maturitas*, an English-language European medical journal.

The author, Dr. Marc L'Hermite, found that five to seven percent of women on conjugated equine estrogens could get severe high blood pressure and that they would return to normal when the hormone-replacement therapy was withdrawn. A bibliographic reference to this article also appeared in Dr. Lonnie Barbach's book *The Pause*. Not one physician at my HMO had mentioned these concerns.

To obtain more information about what alternative health solutions were available and how particular products would change my body or health, I searched the Web under the keywords "menopause," "alternative healthcare," "herbs," "homeopathy," and "naturopathy." I also looked under "natural progesterone."

Through this search I found the *Meno Times*, a quarterly journal published in San Rafael, Calif. I subscribed because it had the information I sought on Dr. John Lee's book *Natural Progesterone: The Multiple Roles of a Remarkable Hormone*.

Also through my search I found a laboratory that would test my saliva and tell me whether my hormones were balanced. Most of all, I wanted to know how taking natural progesterone would affect my fast thyroid and adrenaline-drenched body, with its low blood sugar and excess insulin production.

My HMO physicians did not answer these questions, but told me that going off conjugated equine estrogen and synthetic progestin was like a diabetic going off insulin. On the Net I found physicians who answered my letters, labs that sold natural progesterone cream that I could use to prevent bone loss after menopause, and other labs that could monitor my condition until I found a doctor in my community who would listen to alternative solutions to menopausal questions.

I even found the Menopause Matters page created by Susan Czernicka, who said she "learned about herbal treatment of menopause when there were too few resources available to help her with her many symptoms and too few medical providers with open minds." She will answer questions sent to her at susan270@world.std.com.

For those who don't have Web access, there is the Menopause mailing list. To subscribe, send e-mail to listserv@ psuhmc.hmc.psu.edu with **subscribe menopaus *Your Name*** in the message body. (The list spells 'menopaus' without an 'e.')

The "black cohosh" that I mentioned in my letter to the **alt.support.menopause** newsgroup is an estrogenic herb and vasodilator, and I wanted to find out how safe it was and whether it was as good for menopause as the homeopaths and naturopaths claimed, as well as how much to use and what effects it would have. I found the **alt. folklore.herbs** newsgroup helpful, as well as articles by Anthony Brook entitled "Why Herbs?" and "Historic Uses of Herbs" at the <u>Drum Holistic Herbs</u> page. I also read studies that black cohosh had a possible effect on the heart rhythm. I didn't want to take a chance with black cohosh because the results I had read didn't arrive at a conclusion as to how black cohosh actually changed or otherwise affected heart rhythms.

I wanted to find out everything I could about natural progesterone, so I went to the Health and Science page at <u>Polaris Network</u>, http://www.polaris.net/~health/ which described itself as "A Guide to Understanding and Controlling PMS, Fertility, Menopause, and Osteoporosis." It contained information about natural progesterone and how it balances the side effects of unopposed estrogen, how it's required for proper thyroid function and progestin counterparts in the drug industry.

It also offered a seemingly sound scientific and unbiased evaluation of how certain hormones affect the system, what the hormone's results are on various bodily functions, and side effects. And it had an excellent bibliography of books and medical journal articles on osteoporosis reversal using natural progesterone.

I wanted to query a physician about the high blood pressure resulting from the equine oral estrogen I was taking, and at the <u>Atlanta Reproductive Health Centre</u> page I was able to send e-mail to a doctor who answered my question quickly, providing information that I could consider when making my final decisions or in looking further. His answer was more to the point than the counseling I had received from my own physician.

Another doctor of mine had wanted to give me high blood pressure medicine on top of the estrogen and synthetic progestin. I asked him to consider the alternative—taking me off the hormones to see whether a low-salt diet and exercise could change things—because before I went on hormones my blood pressure wasn't high.

The Internet became one of my best alternative healthcare information resources after the last of three reproductive endocrinologists I saw (not affiliated with my HMO) told me to wait two months to see how I felt off the hormones.

Menopause is a mega-business. More than 100 books a year fill the store shelves on this subject and more than 3,500 baby boomers enter menopause daily. This captivated audience represents a huge market for makers of hormones, vitamins, and other specialty products, much of which is advertised on the Web. So a wealth of information has appeared on the Internet to meet the needs of the 38- to 55-year-olds undergoing menopause, as well as younger women with PMS, infertility, and contraception concerns.

Another resource I found informative was the Women's Health Hot Line newsletter. Its topics include infertility, endometriosis, contraception, sexually transmitted diseases, stress, menopause, and PMS. Most of all, it doesn't close its pages to alternative therapies for women who can't tolerate standard hormone replacement therapy.

Hernia Hunt

This year my husband needed hernia repair surgery, but his busy HMO surgeon spent only a very short time briefing him a month before his surgery. Because it would take hours to describe in detail what is done during hernia repair surgery, he searched on the topic using Web search engines, which yielded a list of information about all kinds of hernias.

The most thorough site discovered was the Hernia Information Home Page in England. It included articles that explained such things as the benefits of using mesh rather than stitches to close incisions. Information about hiatal hernias and diaphragmatic hernias could be found at the Collaborative Hypertext of Radiology. There was more information about hernias on the Net than my husband could possibly find time to read.

After seeing shark cartilage in many health food stores, my husband asked his surgeon about its ability to aid in faster wound-healing. The surgeon laughed, yet I found several references to articles discussing shark cartilage on the Internet. Some medical journal articles on the healing and other properties and uses of shark cartilage can be found on the Simone Protective Pharmaceuticals page. Also at the site I found health-style questionnaires, in-depth descriptions of a variety of nutrient products, and how each product affects the body. You'll also find information about where to order or buy shark cartilage from pharmacists.

Search Tips

From the many healthcare sites I visited, my three-ring binder is packed with more than 500 pages of answers to questions. Productive keyword searches can be made using terms such as "alternative health," "healthcare," "medical," "medicine," "nurses," "nutrition," "pharmacy," "physicians," and "smart drugs." I found the search word "healthcare" to be more specific for asking personal medical questions than trying to search under the word "health."

Some sites are best reached through links on dedicated healthcare Web pages. For example, Subhas Roy has a created a page with links to 25 other Internet health sites at <u>Health Info</u>. There also is a large collection of links at the <u>Internet Medical and Mental Health Resources</u> page. It's maintained by Jeanine Wade, Ph.D., a licensed psychologist in Austin, Texas. One particularly comprehensive directory of health and medical sites on the Web is <u>MedWeb</u>, which lists Web sites and mailing lists in 70 categories, from AIDS to toxicology.

One of the best medical referral Web sites I found was <u>Richard C. Bowyer's</u> page. (You'll find it when you scroll past all his genealogy information.) Bowyer's page has links to numerous sites, such as U.S. hospitals, medical resources, medical journals, medical schools, medical students, medico legal resources, oncology, pathology, and different surgical disciplines, such as plastic surgery, general surgery, laparoscopic surgery, and telesurgery. Healthcare workers of all specializations also can find job opportunities on some of these sites.

My son, a neuroradiologist (physician), was interested in <u>Medline</u>, a collection of medical and scientific reports used by physicians, articles on the educational needs of physicians and the public, physicians' supplies, prescriptions, and advice by pharmacists about drugs. Clinical cancer information that is intended for physicians is useful to patients as well. There is a listing of surgeons according to the types of surgery they perform, the notes of the Physician Reliance Network, and a Gopher menu of physicians listed according to their specialty.

As for informative newsletters available on the Net, I highly recommend the <u>University Of California At Berkeley Wellness Letter At The Electronic Newsstand</u>. It contains the latest news of preventive medicine and practical advice—including information on nutrition, weight control, self-care, prevention of cancer and heart disease, exercise, and dental care.

As a medical journalist, I found the Journal of the American Medical Association (JAMA) to be a reliable resource. If you are looking for a description of a particular drug, the Physician's GenRx Web site provides a database of drugs you can search. You must register first.

In seeking answers to my health questions, I found the Internet to be a valuable source for a wide range of healthcare information. I'm sure your efforts will be rewarded, too.

Selected Health Sites

Anesthesiology & Surgery Center *Offers travel warnings and immunization, medical dictionary.*
Cancer Related Links *Facts, figures, prevention.*
Harvard Medical Gopher *Harvard publications, access to the Countway Library's online catalog (HOLLIS), and medicine.*
Health Letter on the CDC
Health on the Internet Newsletter *Links to NewsPages, CNN Food & Health, MEDwire, describes new health-related Web sites, topic of the month.*
HyperDOC *Sponsored by the National Library of Medicine.*
LifeNet *Positive thinking and right-to-life point of views. Discussion about euthanasia.*
The Mayo Clinic *tour of the Mayo clinic; description of programs.*
Med Help International *Provides medical information about many illnesses. Treatment is described in layman's terms.*
Mednews *A biweekly newsletter that welcomes submissions.*
Medical Information Resource Center *Lists and a referral directory.*
Medicine OnLine *Career-related educational content and discussion groups.*
Medscape *For health professionals and consumers. Bulletin boards and a quiz testing your knowledge of surgery. Registration required.*
The National Organization of Physicians Who Care *Nonprofit organization ensuring quality healthcare. Newsletters, articles about Medicare reform and HMOs.*
OncoLink, the University of Pennsylvania Cancer Resource *Thorough information about pediatric and adult cancers.*
Physicians Guide to the Internet *For new physicians.*
Robert Wood Johnson Foundation Gopher *Biological archives at Indiana university, molecular biology database, NYU Medical Gopher.*

Chapter Four

Nutritional Genomics
for the Consumer

How are you managing your gene expression? In what direction are you moving? How do you make more intelligent *choices* of food to *nourish* your individual *genotype*? What is meant by *intelligent foods* that target and nourish *specific* genes?

Clinical dieticians and nutritionists, by allying with molecular geneticists, genetics counselors, physicians, molecular *genealogists*, family historians, phenomics professionals, nutritional and medical anthropologists, and archaeogeneticists are *collaborating* with consumers of genetics testing, but what are they really *sharing*?

If not so much raw materials such as DNA from donors, is shared, then how about *access* to information—databases and various discussion forums online and e-mailing lists equally open to consumers, licensed healthcare providers, and research scientists? Who controls access to new research—the consumers, the corporations, or the scientists?

Can the average consumer afford to find out what to eat for improved health and nourishment based upon tests of genetic expression? Can consumers *override* any inherited risks revealed in the genetic signature with foods and nutraceuticals individually tailored? What does it mean to eat 'smarter' foods that target specific genes compared to eating more intelligently regarding choice?

Scientists compare genetic distances between populations by comparing the frequencies of forms of genes called 'alleles.' Mutant alleles can be mapped as population genetics markers. Some, but not all mutations in genes may put you at risk for certain chronic diseases if you eat the wrong foods for your genotype. The solution is to eat more 'intelligent' foods customized to your individual genetic profile.

Research also looks at rare alleles. Their rarity gives them special power as markers of genetic similarity. There's a good chance two identical mutant alleles share a common origin. You can map genes for ancestral origin, migrations, or to reveal risks of disease depending upon which genes you map.

This book is for beginners with no science background. It's a consumer's guide book to nutritional genomics—genetic testing and profiling for foods tailored to your genotype and ancestry. The chapters also are about how to interpret DNA testing for family history and ancestry.

How do you as a consumer, not a scientist, choose the smartest food tailored to your genetic signature? How do you interpret your DNA test results for ancestry or family history? What is the *link* between tailoring your foods to your genetic expression and tracing your ancestry though DNA testing? And what genes are tested for either reason? How do you bridge the gap between nutritional genomics profiling and testing DNA for deep ancestral origins?

Does ethnicity play any role in tailoring your food and nutraceuticals, drug dosages, or healthcare? How much can the average consumer self-educate and/or start a private DNA bank for a consumer or patient group? How do you raise funds, contract with research scientists, and form or serve groups needing their DNA researched for specific reasons? How does learning how to interpret the results of your DNA tests for ancestry relate to understanding genetic tests for cardiovascular or other inheritable risks?

Start researching on your own what you need to know as a consumer to have more *choices* in customizing foods for your genetic signature—your genotype. What are some realistic applications of genetic testing and profiling?

This book will lead you to find out more about taking control of what happens to DNA that you may donate for research. You'll find out how to be in charge of your own nourishment and nutrition. Genetic profiling helps you to customize what you eat. How do you nourish your body? What can your genes reveal to you through genetic testing and profiling? It's your private information and should remain private. A good place to release it finally would be in a time capsule and history scrapbook for your heirs. Here are how some branches of human genetic history are linked to your nutrition, ancestry, and most of all nourishment.

Prosopography is all about human history and genes that travel because your genes have both a cultural and a biological component. The cultural component includes onomastics which is the study of the origin of a name and its geographical and historical utilization. Proteomics is about drug discovery. Pharmacogenetics researches how your genes respond to various drugs and dosages to avoid adverse reactions to medicines. Nutrigenomics (nutritional genomics) brings together nutrition and genetics.

Put all these branches of molecular genetics together with molecular geneal-ogy. Add nutritional genomics—molecular nutrition, and what do you have? Knowledge of how every molecule in your body responds to certain foods, lifestyles or exercise can now be studied at the molecular level. New sciences such as pharmacogenetics open doors to learning how your genes respond to nutrition and nourishment. Maybe you want to know how your body responds to certain herbs, nutraceuticals (supplements), foods, or any chemical in your environment, even a skin lubricant or salve or a cosmetic. It's all within the sciences of pharma-cogenetics and/or nutrigenomics. Today, it's not just about how your body responds. You look at the molecular level, the cellular level to study how your genes respond to nourishment, medicine, lifestyle, and the environment.

What if you take many prescription drugs and want to know how rapidly or slowly your body is metabolizing the medicine? You are concerned about the drugs building up in your body or interacting with one another. Pharmacogenetics tests several of your genes. With food menus, nutrigenomics tests other genes. At least you can find out whether you metabolize fast, slow, or like the majority of people. One size will never fit all people because genes recom-bine. They shuffle, and individuals have different responses to different drugs, cosmetics, or foods.

Multidisciplinary nutrition research and collaboration is necessary for nutri-tional genomics to bring together diverse expertise. Scientists working in the dis-ciplines of nutrition, biochemistry, and genetics need to share, collaborate, and interface in this field. If scientists are more concerned about positioning them-selves first in publishing their research and won't share DNA with all scientists, how can research ever move forward?

You might want to read "The Metabolic Basis of Inherited Disorders," 6th ed. McGraw-Hill, New York: 2649–2680, 1989. Then compare the latest research in nutritional genomics on how smart foods (foods tailored to your genetic signa-ture) influence risk of chronic disease. The longer science studies the entire genome (rather than the specific SNPs for certain chronic diseases) the more information will be forthcoming on how food and lifestyle influence your health based on the genes you inherited.

According to the National Institutes of Health, (See their Web site at: http://www.nigms.nih.gov/funding/htm/yrgenes.html), "Your lifestyle, the food you eat, and where you live and work can all affect how you respond to medi-cines. But another key factor is your DNA, which contains your genes. Scientists are trying to figure out how the make-up of your DNA can contribute to the way you respond to medicines, including pain-killers with codeine like Tylenol®#3, antidepressants like Prozac®, and many blood pressure and asthma medicines.

Scientific discoveries made through this research will provide information to guide doctors in prescribing the right amount of the right medicine for you.

"The National Institutes of Health aims to improve the health of all Americans through medical research that solves mysteries about how the human body normally works—and how and why it doesn't work, when disease occurs. One goal of this research is to help improve the good effects of medicines while preventing bad reactions."

Click on the Web site of the National Institutes of Health at: http://www.nigms.nih.gov/funding/htm/qanda.html to see their question and answer site. The point is that one size doesn't fit all when it comes to medicine or food or even cosmetics and skin products. According to the National Institutes of Health, here is the National Institutes of Health's answer to the question of "Aren't prescribed medicines already safe and effective?"

On their question and answer page, they reply, "For the most part, yes. But medicines are not 'one-size-fits-all.' While typical doses work pretty well for most people, some medicines don't work at all in certain people or the medicines can cause annoying, or even life-threatening, side effects." If you're wondering why one size doesn't fit all since our DNA is supposed to be so similar world-wide, it really varies due to some people's genetic variations, diversity, and mutations.

According to the National Institutes of Health (reprinted here with permission) from their Web site at: http://www.nigms.nih.gov/funding/htm/qanda.html#, "As medicines move through the body, they interact with thousands of molecules called proteins. Because each person is genetically unique, we all have tiny differences in these proteins, which can affect the way medicines do their jobs.

"The National Institutes of Health is providing money to scientists at universities and medical centers who come up with the best plans for carrying out research on how people respond differently to medicines. Curing and preventing disease is the National Institutes of Health's highest priority. Research on how people respond differently to medicines will make current and future treatments for diseases such as asthma, diabetes, heart disease, depression, and cancer safer and more effective. A bonus of this type of research will be a better understanding of the role many different genes play in causing or contributing to these and other diseases.

"The National Institutes of Health is providing money to scientists at universities and medical centers who come up with the best plans for carrying out research on how people respond differently to medicines.

"National Institutes of Health-funded scientists at universities and medical centers across the country will recruit volunteers from a wide variety of groups. Research of this type relies upon studying many different people with a broad range of genetic make-ups to find the small, but normal, genetic differences among them.

"Most of these research studies will involve simply rubbing the inside of a volunteer's cheek with a cotton swab. Scientists will then pull out DNA from inside the cheek cells they have collected. There is no health risks associated with this type of test."

"The first benefits to patients could come as soon as a few years from now. From then on, the knowledge gained through this type of research is expected to help doctors tailor the medicines they prescribe to best suit each patient's individual needs."

So what can the consumer do now to benefit as soon as possible from genetic testing? How can you apply the DNA test results to changing your lifestyle now in order to improve your well-being? Education is out there, and much of it is available free on the Web and in scientific journals available at most medical school libraries open to the public. How do you screen the information?

Foods Tailored to Your Genotype

How do your genes respond to what you eat? How many diet-by-DNA book titles are there? Books on smarter foods? Tailored menus? Extracts of plants? DNA tests for ancestry? Ancestry and eating? According to Dr. Fredric D. Abramson, PhD, S.M., President and CEO of *AlphaGenics, Inc.*, Genes are distributed, function, and work in such ways that nearly every reasonable diet could work well in about six percent of the population.

Are you eating smart foods—foods tailored to your genotype—DNA, your ancestry, and your entire genome of genes? Are you ready to get a picture of your response to your nutrition? How can you eat to nourish your genotype? According to Genomics 120, a science, nutrition, and health Web site at: http://g120.com/products/genomicscience.html, are you wondering why in the United States currently only 50,000 people out of some 280 million live to be even 100 years old, or that your body may be aging nearly twice the rate it should be because you're eating the wrong food for your genetic signature?

There is a strong connection between nutrition and genotype, especially in regards to your cardiovascular and central nervous system health. So you need to tailor foods intelligently to your genetic expression. The media buzz about 'intelligent' foods or 'smart' foods really means eating clean, safe, whole foods based on what your individual genes need to thrive. Not all your genes are tested. You might start your food research at the Web site of Food Resource, a source of science-based and business savvy information for the food industry at: http://food.oregonstate.edu/nutri.html.

What happens when diet books for your condition aren't working for you? Maybe salt restriction isn't working but exercise is for your condition. How do your genes respond to nutrition and *nourishment*? Are your genes intelligent, conscious, and communicating with you about their nutritional needs? If they are, so are the foods you eat. Your genes interact and collaborate as a team.

The language of communication is written in the human genome, in your individual genetic signature—in your DNA, in particular SNPs, and in all your genes and cellular material. Even your blood type is expressed in all the cells of your body. How does all this information signal you about what 'smart' foods and nutraceuticals to choose in order to help prevent or delay chronic disease for which your genes may put you at risk?

A slogan reads, "Smart foods for intelligent people." Nutritional genomics is a buzz word in the news. Testing DNA for ancestry also bridges gaps in regard to customizing smarter foods to your genotype. Phenomics is about customized healthcare and medicine tailored to your genetic profile. Prosopography is an independent science of social history embracing genealogy, onomastics and demography. If you're interested in metabolic typing, one Web site for Personal Metabolic Typing is at: http://www.wholebodyhealth.us/. Dentists may be interested to know that gum disease is genetic and may be caused by a genetic predisposition to diabetes, heart disease, or low birth weight. A genetic profile on patients with deep pockets of gum disease might be useful. Check out the Holistic Dental Network at: http://holisticdentalnetwork.com/products_services.php.

Cracking the human genome code is so new and tests so costly. Currently only certain genetic markers are tested. The genetic signatures tested include genes that tell you about risk for certain diseases. Nutritional genomics as a field of research also is abbreviated as a generic term to read 'nutrigenomics.'

Without testing all the genes, how can you know about all the diseases for which you may be at risk? And without knowing all the information that every one of your gene's reveals, how can you develop a plan to override your genetic risks by nourishing your genes with what they need to stay healthier? **Here is how some scientists answered these questions.**

According to Dr. Fredric D. Abramson, PhD, S.M., President and CEO of *AlphaGenics, Inc.*, "The key to using diet to manage genes and health lies in managing gene expression (which we call the Expressitype). Knowing your genotype merely tells you a starting point. Genotype is like knowing where the entrance ramps to an interstate can be found. They are important to know, but tell you absolutely nothing about what direction to travel or how the journey will go. That is why Expressitype must be the focus." You can contact AlphaGenics, Inc. at: http:// www.Alpha-Genics.com or write to: Maryland Technology Incubator, 9700 Great Seneca Highway, Rockville, MD 20850.

Alpha Genics, Inc. is a nutrigenomics science company. A sidebar on the company's Web site from Dr. Fredric Abramson, CEO reads (reprinted here with permission), "We are about to see a revolution in our concept of diet. Each of us is a unique organism and for the first time in human history, genetic research is confirming that one diet is not optimum for everyone.

Science is discovering that each individual's DNA processes food and nutritious supplements in a unique way. Through the development of a cutting-edge DNA analytical system and consumer guidance, Alpha Genics will be able to tune nutrition to meet the needs of each individual resulting in optimum health, peak performance, and enhanced creativity." What I also like about Alpha-Genics Inc. is that they have an independent, separate Ethics Board. Check out that Web site at: http://www.alpha-genics.com/ethics_board.php.

It is not part of the regular Board of Directors. It has five members: three outsiders, one representative from the Board of Directors, and one representative of the employees. The Ethics Board has no veto power, but has a seat on the Board of Directors. Compensation for the Ethics Board members comes through a blind trust, which means the Ethics Board has neither control nor knowledge of how the funds develop.

"I created this because I think companies need to have independent voices to provide reality checks," says Dr. Fredric Abramson. "It is something like that scene in Patton when he talks about the Roman conqueror returning home to glory, with someone standing just beside him reminding him that fame is fleeting. An independent Ethics Board helps us make better choices."

Consumers can bridge the gap between ethics boards and the media by acting as liaisons, ombudsmen, lobbyists, trustees, recruiters, communicators, independent board members, fee-for-service contractors, industry watchers, or volunteers. Get involved in the nutritional genomics industry.

You even can put together corporate gift baskets full of nutritional genomics products or samples. Throw a nutritional genomics party in any home, office, or meeting pace, in church basements, teacher's lounges after school, or at conventions. Make tape recordings about nutritional genomics and post the radio-length broadcasts to your Web site. So many news stories in the media give the impression that the average consumer will have to *wait a decade* for genomic testing to be applied to customized foods.

For example, the New York Times Magazine published an article by NY Times Magazine writer Bruce Grierson titled, "What Your Genes Want You to Eat: New Way to Look at Disease." The article also appeared in the Sacramento Bee, a daily newspaper, on Sunday July 13, 2003 on the Science page. Sundays are great for reading the Science page in the Forum section. There's time to read the cutting-edge science articles, many of which are reprinted from other, major urban publications. It's a family tradition for four decades.

I was impressed by the media buzz around the relatively new field of nutritional genomics. Last year the media buzz circled around testing DNA for ancient ancestry and genealogy, during which I took several DNA tests for ancestry and enjoyed the results. This year DNA and diet is fast-track news. DNA and foods also tie into food safety and security issues.

I like to know that when I go into a health food store and buy a package of imported powdered ginger under the title of herbs or botanicals that it's clean and contains no toxic pesticides, residues, bad bacteria, or unsafe chemicals. I often thought about who inspects these imports and do they rush through, take enough time, or have enough staff? If I buy fresh ginger root, I'm concerned whether it's organic or still full of pesticide residue. On the other hand, who has time to think these thoughts?

It all came rushing back when I went into a health food store last month, walked past an open bin where a child about twelve years old had just put her hand into the couscous, grabbed a fist full of the grain-like pasta, tossed it into her mouth, chewed it, spit it back into her palm and replaced the couscous that she had just spit into her hand, back into the bin with the rest of the grain. Her mother was busy looking at other products.

She didn't realize I was standing beside her ready to take a scoop myself of the oat groats in the next bin. The scoop hit the floor, and she picked it up and replaced it. The cashier was in the front of the store, the manager in the back room. Why couldn't the store change the bins so that nobody else could spit into the grain? When I brought this to the cashier's attention, she shrugged, looked down, and acted as if nothing had happened. I wondered at that instant, if this is how one consumer's word is received, how will the public perceive us?

There's power in numbers, in grouping together. I wished I had my video camera at that moment. There's also power in the media—the reputable, credible media that bridges gaps between science and the public. It's time for some consumers to become "media people." Let's watch the watchers and look at the media.

The article titled, "What Your Genes Want You to Eat: New Way to Look at Disease," had its first opening sentence beginning with a trip to the "'diet doc' circa 2013." I eagerly wanted this kind of testing to be available now, not in 2013. So I turned to Dr. Frederic Abramson, CEO of Alpha-Genics Incorporated to interview by email on his views. Dr. Abramson also teaches part-time at Johns Hopkins University, in the graduate program in Biotechnology.

I asked Dr. Frederic Abramson, CEO of Alpha-Genics Incorporated the following questions in an October 2004 e-interview. Here are his answers.

1. When do you think genomic testing might be available to most consumers?

This is an important question. From a practical perspective, genomic testing—for part of a person's total genome—is possible today. We can test for several thousand genes right now. So this leads to two sub-questions: When will testing of an entire genome become possible? When will low-cost testing be available?

Experts argue about whether we have 30,000 or 70,000 genes, or somewhere in between. Regardless of the number, we are five years away from a comprehensive full genotype test of all genes in a person. By genotype, I mean the identification of which genes a person has.

But it is not your genotype which determines things. It is the work that your specific genes do. Think of genotype as the location of exit ramps on an interstate. You need to know where these are, but they tell you nothing about where you are going and what the journey will be like.

To identify these, we must look at each gene's level of activity, called "gene expression." We call the gene expression the Expressitype. Gene expression changes over time for many genes. How do we know this? Because we age. We start as children, go though puberty, become adults, and then start declining. All of this is substantially under genetic control. Some people age faster than other. It's in their genes.

Right now testing costs a fair amount. And seldom is gene testing covered by insurance. But over time, the technology advances will enable very low cost tests. For example, measuring gene expression in several thousand genes can cost between $800 to $3,000, depending on who does it. But a Japanese company is working on a test that will end up costing less than $100 for 900 genes. Thus, one thing we can be sure of is that the costs will drop. Just like computers, VCR's and microwaves.

We are working to bring the test cost to be under $1,000, with a monthly follow-up of around $79. The monthly fee lets you contact us by phone or email anytime to ask whether something you want to eat might help you or not.

We are working with Carnegie Mellon University in Pittsburgh to develop a small implantable device that will measure vital chemicals in the blood, and send signals outside the body. This will let us track what is happening in a person around the clock, every day, with much more accuracy and less guesswork.

2. What do you think is the most important area of research in nutritional genomics today?

The most important area is to identify how the dietary system, which is composed of hundreds and thousands of chemicals in varying dosages, interacts with the thousands of genes in the genome to produce health, or illness. This is generally called "systems biology." Basically, we can no longer look at single things for easy answers. It won't be just a question of whether you eat blueberries or bananas or rice, but what balance of each of these you eat over time.

This points me to the second area, to understand the dynamics of how changes in diet influence the work each person's genes is doing. The value of systems biology is that ultimately, we will be able to identify individualized responses to diet, based on genetic composition.

3. Do you have any advice for those who are looking for tailored diets for specific conditions—if genotype testing is not available today, what is the next best thing for the average consumer who has already had a DNA test of merely the mtDNA or Y chromosome for ancestry?

Ironically, many of the folk suggestions about diet weren't far wrong. So first look to your family history. If you have heart disease in your family, think about a diet that has a bit less fat and more antioxidants. There are similar observations about other conditions like arthritis and cancer.

Generally, if you have a DNA test at this point, it is for one or very few genes. This helps. But remember that most major health conditions are the result of many, many genes acting in concert, not just one gene.

I'll admit it can be confusing with so many different recommendations about diet. To me, this reflects the way in which our genetic diversity makes one diet work well for me and not well for you, while another diet has the exact opposite effect.

4. What is the area of research your company is focusing on now?

Our research focus is to understand how the specific ingredients of diet influence genetic activity. And by diet we include food, supplements, medications, chemicals in water, and even cosmetics, for all of these contain chemicals that influence genes.

The goal of our research is to translate the science into practical day-to-day advice for each person, based on his/her own genetic profile and genetic activity.

We want to make genomics something that is useful for each of use every day instead of some industrial science.

This is the same thing that happened when Edison invented the light bulb. Suddenly, electricity was something that every home needed. For us, our success in delivering NutriGenomics to the consumer will make genomics something that everyone will want to use to live their lives a bit better.

5. Where can I refer readers today to learn more?

The amount of literature on the Internet is growing almost daily. Two weeks ago, the commission of the FDA mentioned NutriGenomics in his major speech at Harvard.

We welcome readers to contact us. We are assembling the world's first comprehensive NutriGenomic knowledge base, which we will use to help consumers make better choices. We build our research insights on the actual experience of what real people do.

Our current high priority is a totally new method to prevent viral infections using NutriGenomics. We discovered this in January, and have been working to get government support to conduct this important research. We believe we can develop a way to protect many people from the dangers of certain types of viruses, such as a weaponized flu.

6. Do you work with patients directly or only with their managing physicians or both?

We will work with patients directly and with physicians. When a physician is involved, we will be sure to include the physician in the information loop so the person continues to get the best care.

7. How many genes do you test? Do you prescribe a diet or nutraceuticals based on the results?

In the current stage, we will test about 2,000 genes, mainly for the cardiovascular cluster (cardiovascular disease, diabetes, obesity, hypertension, high cholesterol). The virus testing is planned to be a separate test.

The specific food/supplement recommendations are made directly to the person. These change as the person's genetic activity changes. It would be a mistake to prescribe one type of diet for life. Our genes and bodies don't work that way.

The procedure is simple. We get a sample from you, typically from your cheek lining or blood (if you go to a physician). We identify the genes (genotype) and the amount of genetic activity for each gene (expressitype). We provide you a report summarizing the results. Then, depending on your decision, we will provide you general dietary recommendations based on your genes, or will begin to work with you as often as daily to help you choose what you like to eat.

It is worth noting here that the so-called 'med diet' is based on a month of eating, whereas the USDA model is a daily model. We prefer the monthly approach for the evidence is that eating has a cumulative effect. Another way of saying this is "no one meal will ever hurt you. It is the combination of lots of bad meals that hurts. So knock yourself out."

Fredric D. Abramson, Ph.D., S.M.
President & CEO
AlphaGenics, Inc.
http://www.Alpha-Genics.com

According to Dr. Fredric D. Abramson, PhD, S.M., Esq. President and CEO of AlphaGenics, Inc., our genes determine how we respond to our environment. In the industry, nutritional genomics also is abbreviated as 'nutrigenomics.' Let's look at Dr. Abramson's article below titled: *"About NutriGenomics,"* Copyright 2002, 2003. Reprinted here with permission.

About NutriGenomics

Fredric Abramson, Ph.D., S.M., Esq.
Copyright 2002, 2003

Our genes determine who we are, how we develop and age, and how we respond to our environment. They are the blueprints that define our potential. But they do not act in a vacuum. They respond to and actually help shape our environment. That environment includes what we put into our body in food, water, supplements, nutraceuticals and pharmaceuticals.

Together, our genes and environment control our health and our susceptibility to disease. NutriGenomics involves decoding how the molecular composition of our diet, which includes food, supplements, pharmaceuticals and water) influences the work being done by our genes, and then defining personalized dietary strategies to tune each person's gene expression pattern, called the "Expressitype." This tuning process must be changed dynamically as the person's genetic activity changes.

"NutriGenomics lets people pick the foods they eat based on how well the foods make their genes function."

Because what we eat influences our health and the way our genes work, we have the opportunity to let people control their health destiny in a whole new way. This is what NutriGenomics is about: calibrating the mix and amounts of what ingredients we put into our body so that our genes work at their best, for our best health status. By building on each person's genetic uniqueness, NutriGenomics focuses on what that individual's genes are doing and how that person can pick and choose things from their environment that will make his/her genes work better or worse.

AlphaGenics approach is to identify what parts of your diet are making your genes work badly, and determine the best mixture in your diet to calibrate and tune the work your genes are doing. Our goal is to adjust your genetic activity, without changing your genes, by dynamically adjusting the mix of what you put into your body as your body changes over time.

Basic Terms

> ▶ Genotype: The entire set of genes of an individual.
> ▶ Expressitype: The profile of gene expression activity in an individual at a moment in time.
> ▶ Phenotype: The observable characteristics of an individual.
> ▶ NutriGenomics: The science that relates how the molecular inputs from a person's environment influence and control gene expression.
> ▶ Qwink: A molecule or particle in the environment that can change gene expression directly or indirectly.
> ▶ Expressitype Knowledge Transfer System: A proprietary information/ knowledge management system that integrates individual longitudinal data with a variety of scientifically verified data elements. Its outputs include personalized, dynamic dietary strategies as well as a variety of scientific and research-oriented solutions.

Our dietary environment influences how our genes work

Many different ingredients exist in a person's dietary environment. They exist as both natural molecules and artificial compounds and are found in food as well as in our water, and in dietary supplements, cosmetics and medications. Even in the air we breathe. Some are present by design; others as a by-product. So, for example, the common tomato is known to have over 300 different natural molecules. Some ingredients are man-made, but most are natural substances whose variety and health-effects are not even fully explored.

The key to NutriGenomics is identifying how specific compounds or chemicals in our diet influence the activity of one or more genes, and hence our health.

Our focus is on our genetic activity (Expressitype) and not just what genes we have (Genotype). Knowing your genotype is a lot like knowing where the entrance is to an interstate highway. It is very useful and important, but it doesn't tell you what direction to go in or when you will be able to stop for gas.

The term "Qwink" was coined to refer to any molecule in the dietary stream that influences gene expression. Qwinks are found in foods, supplements, cosmetics, water and pharmaceutical compounds. They include basic ingredients such as sugars, proteins and fat as well as very specialized substances such as vitamins or toxins. A Qwink may be a natural substance or synthetic.

A Qwink is neutral as to whether it has a positive or negative effect. If the gene expression moves in the direction to provide better health or reduce risk, it is good; if it moves to worsen a person's health status, it is bad. Thus, it is only the effects that are good or bad. For example, a pesticide residue that survives in the food chain and influences gene expression is a Qwink.

While pesticides are generally considered harmful, interestingly enough, there is some evidence that certain pesticides could actually reduce the risk of cancer, at least in model systems.[1]

NutriGenomics calibrates dietary inputs and patterns to provide different Qwink types and concentrations to the genetic machinery.

The impact of a Qwink typically depends on its concentration and dosage frequency.

One of the amazing aspects of human biology is that it responds differently to varied Qwink concentrations. Take arsenic, for example. Most people know that arsenic in high doses can kill. What is less commonly known, however, is that at very low concentrations, arsenic is considered a nutrient.

The same will be found for how Qwinks work. At very low concentrations, one set of genes may be affected while a much higher concentration may change expression in an entirely different set of genes.

NutriGenomics is personalized genomics

The way a person's dietary environment influences gene expression and health is called NutriGenomics. NutriGenomics is a scientific platform that permits focused personalized adjustments to a person's dietary environment. An advantage of NutriGenomics is that it is a unifying standard that includes the effect of dietary supplements, nutraceuticals, pharmaceuticals and cosmetics in addition to what a person normally eats, as well as environmental factors such as toxins, contaminants and infectious agents, such as viruses and bacteria. The scientific goal is to identify molecular levers coming from a person's environment that can

---

[1.] John Milner, National Cancer Institute, personal communication, January 2003.

move the person's gene expression patterns in an appropriate direction, and to further identify environmental adjustments that can help improve the person's health status through changes in gene expression.

Our core scientific proposition is that evaluating and modulating a person's Expressitype as it dynamically changes over time is a more potent and acceptable way to prevent and control disease than working with genotype alone. The practical difference between focusing on genotype versus expressitype is comparable to the difference between buying a car based on what Consumer Reports says is its repair frequency and listening to your car coughing and sputtering when you are driving down the highway.

The cycle begins with a person's environment, which interacts with the person's genotype and can up-regulate or down-regulate various genes. The gene expression pattern, the expressitype, in turn, works to produce proteins and otherwise control the person's metabolism and physiology to produce the phenotype. It is a person's phenotype at which we observe health and illness. Examples of phenotype include eye color, blood groups, and various chronic and acute diseases. A person's phenotype in turn helps shape the environment. For example, phenotype can influence what a person chooses to eat. A person who doesn't feel well may eat differently; a person who changes their physical activity may also change how they eat; and so on.

AlphaGenics designed its research and intervention around this cycle. By capturing data and information from each individual, including serial measures of expressitype, and blending this data with scientific knowledge from genomics, nutrition, pharmacology, toxicology, and medicine, we can focus on unraveling the systems biology map of how the complex environment interacts with and influences the comparably complex genome.

Our genome works as a system that takes us through our life cycle

Our genetic apparatus is a complex system designed to sustain our lives in intimate communication with the environment, from birth through puberty and the gradual aging process leading to the end of our lives. It is this complexity that has made it so difficult to find cures or treatments for so many diseases like cancer and heart disease. It is this same complexity that explains why a drug will work in one person, be ineffective in another, and harm a third. It is this complexity that confirms why different people need entirely different diets to lose weight, for example.

The fact is also that almost all of the major health conditions that concerns society today—cancer, heart disease, diabetes, obesity, neurological and similar disorders are all multifactorial and polygenic. Multifactorial means that it is both environment and genetics in combination that explains when, why and where different diseases occur. Polygenic means that multiple genes are involved, not just one.

Three specific aspects of this complexity are worth exploring. First, the number of different genes involved with each of the diseases that plague us can be in the hundreds or even thousands. Second, virtually every chemical that we put into our body influences some genes. And third, our genes typically work collaboratively, where one influences another. Our genes work as an integrated, cohesive system.

A change in gene expression is not always a benefit

The goal of NutriGenomics is to move gene expression patterns to some "best" state. However, because the human genome is complex, an important issue is that an "increase or a decrease" in gene expression is not "always" linked with a benefit. A lot may depend on what the other genes involved are doing as well.

Many different genes are involved in the common health conditions

Most of the common conditions that concern our health are polygenic, i.e. involve many different genes as mentioned above. The goal of the Human Genome Project was to identify thousands of genes and to link these genes to specific health effects. Scientists are also pinpointing exactly where each of these genes are located, or "mapped," on our chromosomes.[2]

Some examples include breast cancer (over 200 genes, 39 of which are mapped to 17 different chromosomes), obesity (over 200 genes; 15 mapped to 11 chromosomes); Diabetes (60 mapped genes to 17 different chromosomes); Lymphoma (200 mapped genes on 22 chromosomes); and hypertension (19 genes on 10 chromosomes).[3]

Qwinks impact multiple genes, not just one

What we put into our body typically influences more than one gene. For example, the natural compound retinoic acid can change expression in more than 500 different genes[4] while the enzyme Cofactor Q10 will up-or down-regulate over 100 different genes.[5]

---

[2] Humans have 22 pairs of chromosomes plus the X and Y.

[3] Obtained from the Human Genome Project web site.

[4] Balmer and Blomhoff, Gene Expression Regulation by Retinoic Acid, Journal of Lipid Research, Vol. 43, 1773–1808 (November 2002).

[5] Linnane AW, et al. Cellular redox activity of CoQ10:effect of Q10 supple. On human skel. muscle. Free Rad Res 2002;36(4):445–453.

Genes work together as a coherent system, not as independent actions.

For a polygenic condition, it is important to realize that the genes involved do not work by themselves but work in a coherent, structured system. We can take as an example the more than 200 different genes implicated in obesity. If each of these genes worked independently of one another, there would be 2 to the 200th power different combinations. This is 1.6 times ten to the 60th power; that is, 1.6 followed by 60 zeros. This number, 1.6 times ten to the 60th, is very large. In fact, it is larger than all the humans who have ever lived on the earth. It is larger than all the organisms, including viruses that have ever lived on the earth.

So clearly, just by observing that different groups or types exist in obesity, one realizes that these 200 genes don't work independently. In fact, what must happen is that when one gene turns on, it in turn regulates ten or twenty others. This interaction among our genes leads to a relatively small, countable number of combinations of gene activity. Instead of the astronomic number calculated above, we have only 100's or 1000's of combinations for this example of obesity. These combinations are the "typical" patterns of gene activation, so to speak the molecular bar codes, each of which could be associated with a form of the disease.

So it is possible to imagine two type of obese people, one with five obesity genes turned on, say numbers 1, 50, 95, 150 and 200, and the rest turned off; the second with twelve different obesity genes turned on. These two different combinations could translate into different obesity effects, where one type of person gains weight easier than the other on the same diet.

While our genes are fixed at birth, the work they do changes as we age

Each person is born with genes they inherited from their parents. The identity of your genes is called the "Genotype." The Genotype is a person's unique collection of genes. Classic genetics described genotypes for hair and eye color, and blood types. For all practical purposes, the genotype is fixed when your parents' sperm and egg unite.

Genes are dynamic engines. Their work varies depending on circumstances and time. The entire genomic system changes its work, as illustrated by the aging process that begins with infancy, moves through childhood, puberty and adulthood, and then to senescence. These genetic mechanisms are starting to be understood.

An example of gradual, almost invisible changes in genetic activity is observed in how menstrual cycles shorten as a woman ages. Research done at the University of Minnesota in the 40's shows that a 40 year old woman has one more menstrual period a year than a 20 year old, and that the one-day per year change in cycle length is linear from 20 to 40. This gradual change suggests that key genetic components to target in NutriGenomics are genes whose activity undergoes very gradual changes over a long time period. This further suggests that many key NutriGenomic interventions will be based on cumulative effects.

It's Gene Expression (Expressitype) Which is Key

The accomplishments of the Human Genome Project mean we will soon be able to identify every gene in a person, in effect, that person's genetic blueprint. Some of these genes will indicate greater risks for certain diseases; other genes will mean less risk than average. An example is the BRCA1 gene for breast cancer. Women with BRCA1 have a significantly higher risk of developing breast cancer than those without it.

The genotype, however, is only a starting place to understand what our genetic destiny might be. This is because the work a gene does is likely to change over time, both according to preprogrammed rules, and in response to environmental influences, notably our food. Some genes are turned on early in life, say during pregnancy, and are switched off permanently. Other genes may just sit there waiting to be activated or to become phenotypically manifest. This appears to be the case with certain diseases that arise later in life, such as Huntington's chorea, a single dominant gene disorder that shows itself in a person's 50's.

Further complicating the situation is that when a gene is "on" it may be operating at one activity level one day and a higher or lower level the next day. A gene's activity is exhibited as "genetic expression," a term that refers to the gene producing RNA and otherwise interacting with a person's metabolism and physiology.

Let's call, in analogy to Genotype, the entire profile of expression of each gene throughout the genome, the "Expressitype." Thus, for any health condition, each person has his or her own Expressitype. The Expressitype is the actual amount of genetic activity produced by each gene that is implicated in or related to a specific health status or condition.

Since for any particular gene that is turned on, the expression level may be changing over time, and because the gene itself may be turned on or off at a particular point in time, a person's Expressitypes is likely to change.

A person's NutriGenomic profile, then, measures what each gene is doing at a point in time. By stringing together a series of NutriGenomic profiles, it is possible to see whether a gene is changing, the direction a gene is going and how fast it is getting there.

The gene-environment interaction is very powerful

The interaction between genes and environment is undisputed. Part of the environment is dietary—what we eat. Another part is lifestyle—how we live our everyday lives. Figure 1 is a general overview of NutriGenomics, starting with the dietary inputs at the base and moving through the genome to the end result of health or illness.

Even well defined genetic disorders respond to environment differences. For example, if identical twins each have the single dominant gene for Huntington's chorea, and the twins have different dietary and exercise programs, the onset of Huntington's chorea can be delayed up to eight years in one of the twins.

Diet has been shown to alter gene expression in several ways Qwinks can act on how DNA is transcribed into RNA They can be involved in various metabolic pathways and can increase or decrease the concentrations of other materials needed by the genome. In other words, Qwink effects can be direct, by changing gene activity itself, or indirect by shifting what is available for the gene to use.

Foods, supplements and other chemical sources are the foundation of NutriGenomics. The ingredients that actively regulate the genome, the Qwinks, can turn genes on and off, and can change the amount of activity for each turned-on gene. The Qwinks help determine the Expressitype, which is the profile of what each gene is doing at a moment in time. Gene expression becomes translated into health, wellness or illness through a person's metabolism and the many proteins in the proteome. Moreover, a person's health status, in turn, influences gene activity and can even change what might be acceptable to eat. An example would be creating an immune response to a certain food (i.e., strawberries) that makes the food dangerous. This system is dynamic, and changes over time as we age and our health changes. Tying these all together are the many biochemical, physiological and metabolic processes with cells and tissues.

*   *   *

Let's profile another company that helps you eat better by revealing disease risks, so your physician can concentrate on focused prevention and treatment tailored to your individual genetic signature. Today, there are companies such as *Genovations*™.

According to Marketing Communications at the North-Carolina-based Great Smokies Diagnostic Laboratory, the company approaches preventive health care by using genetic analysis to provide individuals and their physicians with critical information to more effectively control present and future health. Genovations uses information stored in each person's genes to reveal disease risks and to help each individual lead a healthier life though focused prevention and individualized treatment.

Genes provide the key to a wealth of information unique to each individual that, once unlocked, can serve as a comprehensive guide to a healthier life. By identifying specific genetic risk factors and changes in dietary, lifestyle, nutritional supplements and medications that are most likely to improve each patient's health, Genovations enables physicians to practice truly individualized preventive medicine.

Most consumers will ask about what happens when you go for a genetic test. It's more than the DNA test you might have taken to look at your mtDNA or Y-chromosome for deep ancestry. Instead, the kind of genetic testing you'd take at Genovation, for example is to evaluate specific portions of your genetic code.

Genovations™ testing evaluates specific portions of the genetic code that vary from person to person. These variations are called single nucleotide polymorphisms, or SNPs (pronounced "snips") for short. Everyone has SNPs—they're what make people different from one another—our hair color, our height, our voice, even key aspects of our personality. SNPs are the very seat of our individuality. SNPs also affect our health.

Some SNPs can make people more susceptible or more resistant to common diseases. Others may make the body respond differently to certain diets or lifestyle habits. Read the *Complete Blood Type Diet Encyclopedia.* What nutritional genomics needs is a complete human genome diet dictionary. With 40,000 or more genes in each person shuffling with each generation, individuals inherit different genotypes.

At the same time, some abnormal genes are inherited and make members of some families more at risk than other families. **Here is an e-letter from Kay Patrick, Product Manager, Genovations.**

From: Kay_Patrick
To: 'Anne Hart'
Sent: Tuesday, July 22, 2003 6:46 AM
Subject: RE: Thanks. Just a few questions

Dear Anne:
I have attempted to answer your questions. Please let me know if you have additional questions.

Why are Genovations tests only available through a physician?

Genomic test results are most meaningful and best understood when they are clinically interpreted within the context of a patient's complete health history. For this reason, genomic testing is best managed by a licensed health care professional.

Genovations tests are available only through trained, licensed health care practitioners. Not all practitioners are adequately trained to interpret and use the genomic information revealed in these tests, so Genovations has taken a leading role in providing genomic medical education to health care practitioners.

What does Genovations ™ testing do?

Genovations testing focuses only on SNPs in the genetic code that are associated with common health conditions, such as heart disease, osteoporosis, allergies and asthma, for which simple treatment strategies exist to reduce risk. Testing also evaluates SNPs that affect how each person's body is likely to respond to specific diets, supplements, and medications.

Therapeutic recommendations based upon the genetic results are provided for the practitioner to develop a treatment protocol. In this way, test results can provide the physician with a "road map" for developing a comprehensive, personalized health action plan for each patient.

Example:

Heart Disease

MYTH: All persons with a family history of heart disease can minimize their cardiovascular risk by reducing their dietary intake of fat and salt, exercising more, and taking a cholesterol lowering medication.

REALITY: Heart disease is not simply a condition caused by excess fat and cholesterol. Research has revealed that there are many other modifiable risk factors, some genetically influenced that can predispose a person to heart disease.

For example, some people have a genetic inability to properly metabolize folic acid in the body. This can lead to a build-up of homocysteine in the bloodstream, causing increased risk of blood clots and atherosclerosis. Yet none of the "one-size-fits-all" conventional therapies listed above would reduce this risk. For a person with this genetic variation, the only way to reduce risk is to take the active form of folic acid, which is not found in common vitamin supplements.

High blood pressure is typically treated by restricting an individual's salt intake. However, not all people have the genetic variation (a single nucleotide polymorphism, or SNP-pronounced "snip") that allows them to respond effectively to a salt-restricted diet. Based on their genetic make-up, they may respond better to aerobic exercise. By testing genetic variations, the physician can better identify which therapy is likely to be the most effective for lowering blood pressure in each patient.

Apo E is a protein in the body that affects cholesterol levels. There are three major genetic variations of the Apo E gene that can affect how each person's body breaks down fat and cholesterol in the diet. These three variations can lead to an increased, average, or decreased risk of heart disease. By knowing an individual's Apo E genetic variation, the physician can prescribe the dietary and lifestyle changes, nutritional supplements, or prescription medications most likely to lower cholesterol levels effectively.

What is the process?

Practitioners incorporate genomic testing into their complete work-up along with other phenotypic diagnostic tests. Blood samples are collected in the office, shipped to our laboratory, tested here in our genomics lab and the reported results are shipped back to the ordering practitioner who schedules a follow-up with the patient.

How much does a Genovations test cost?

The cost of Genovations testing depends on the testing option chosen by the patient and the practitioner. The comprehensive testing program, which assesses health risks for a wide range of conditions (including heart disease, osteoporosis, and immune dysfunction) costs about $1,000–$2,000. Focused testing for health risks associated with a single area or condition costs about $300–$500.

Hope that helps.

Sincerely,
Kay Patrick

Product Manager, Genovations
www.genovations.com

*   *   *

An overview of what genes are, how they are inherited, and how many are in the human body is presented on the Web site at: http://www.genovations.com/patient_overview.html.

What Can SNPs Tell You About Your Genotype?

SNPs can even affect whether certain drugs are likely to have severe side effects or not. By evaluating these health-related SNPs, Genovations™ testing allows physicians to develop preventive strategies that are tailored to each patient's unique genetic makeup and health risks. This helps to reduce the guesswork that results from using "one-size-fits-all" approach to preventive medicine.

Genovations™ is a line of tests that is only available for a licensed health care provider (doctor) to order for a patient. The test results are provided directly to the health care provider, who consults with his or her patient. Genovations does not interpret test results for the patient or the health care provider. A patient's health care provider uses the test result information to determine appropriate treatment protocols for the patient. Genovations™ does not provide specific nutriceuticals or supplements recommendations. That is up to the health care provider.

According to marketing communications, "Genovations does not test for SNPs. We currently have 4 profiles that identify specific SNPs related to heart disease, detoxification problems, bone health, and immunology related problems. Each profile identifies between 7 and 15 SNPs." If you want more information about Genovations, write to them, email them, or telephone. Genovations' phone number and email address are listed at its Web site. Since books hang around libraries for years, but phone numbers may or may not change, you can reach Great Smokies Diagnostic Laboratory or Genovations™ as follows: Corporate Headquarters, Great Smokies Diagnostic Laboratory/Genovations™ 63 Zillicoa Street, Asheville, NC 28801, USA

Or go to their Web sites at: http://www.genovations.com/ and/or at: www.gsdl.com. See the Web site at: http://www.gsdl.com/assessments/finddisease/cardiovascular/metabolic_glycemia.html

Read about metabolic glycemia. If you have insulin resistance, or too much insulin pouring out every time you eat certain carbohydrates, you'd want to read more about this and how it changes or affects your arteries and other parts inside your body.

There are excellent sites on the Web to educate yourself before you decide to get tested. Check out your biomarkers. Before you see your doctor, know what questions to ask and what tests to ask for. Then talk it over with your physician.

When you take control over what you eat you are educating yourself as to your body's nutritional requirements to maintain health, stay fit, and prevent or delay chronic illness at any age. Your genetic profile tells you how your genes are responding to the food you eat.

With 30,000, 40,000, or 70,000 genes in each individual and each person inheriting a different genotype, you'd need a customized diet book for each person on Earth.

Each individual's genetic signature is different. Nobody responds exactly the same way to certain foods. That's why genetic testing helps to *customize* food plans for the individual. Some people have allergies. Others respond to foods gradually and silently inside their arteries and organs.

Another buzz word in the media is 'smart' or 'intelligent' foods. It's not that the food is smart or genetically changed. It's that the food in a relatively unprocessed, natural, clean state is free from vermin, full of life and enzymes. That prescribed food according to the person's gene expression is then healthier to eat for that particular person. Another person could be allergic to it and become sicker.

The food itself is freer of toxins. Additionally, the 'smart' or 'intelligent' food terminology really means the act of tailoring or customizing the food to the person's genetic profile. It does not mean the food is genetically altered and may or may not be dangerous to humans. 'Intelligent' foods refer to the results of your genetic testing.

You're the person being smarter by eating what the results of genetic tests reveal. The results are interpreted by a professional. In addition, you need to find out for yourself how to apply the test results to what happens to you when you eat a particular food combination or take a certain group of nutraceuticals. In making a food such as raw soy milk, for example, you need to know that raw soy can take certain nutrients out of your body if the soy milk is not cooked for a certain length of time before it is bottled, cooled and then consumed.

Blue, purple, and red-colored fruit or vegetables are excellent for your health, if your genotype says so. Eating raw blue berries also will take out certain vitamins from your body unless the berries are frozen or cooked.

You need to know how to process raw vegetables and fruits either by cooking and/or freezing before they are consumed so that eating them day after day in certain amounts won't lead to the leaching out of various vitamins, enzymes, or minerals from your body. Knowledge is important here. When you are prescribed certain foods, make sure you know how to prepare them for the maximum nutrient benefits.

Diets need to be tailored to individuals. There are only four blood types, but individual genotypes are different for each person. You'd need a customized diet book for each person on Earth. Each individual's genetic signature is different. Nobody responds exactly the same way to certain foods. That's why genetic testing helps to customize food plans for the individual. Some people have allergies. Others respond to foods gradually and silently inside their arteries and organs.

Not only do people of different ethnicities react differently to the same doses of medicines, but people of different ethnicities react differently to certain foods. It's touchy to bring in the term "race," but studies have found that people of a certain race react differently to certain drugs for certain conditions, and that people of another race react differently to the same dosage given to another race. You can read in medical journal articles for example, on how African Americans respond to glaucoma drugs compared to Caucasian people. You can read about how the same dose of a drug given to an East Asian and a non-East Asian will be too high a dose for the East Asian.

You can read about foods—how people from Northern Europe tolerate milk better than people from Southern Europe, and how people from Southeast Asia hardly tolerate milk at all in many cases. Then, there is always the exception. People are of mixed ancestry. What you need to learn about is the way intelligent foods work with your genes.

You don't know who will react in which ways at the genetic level to the food or medicine or whether the dosage of the drug or the amount of the food will be tolerated or too high or low. Even with varying dosages of nutraceuticals—supplements such as vitamins, food extracts, and minerals, some people benefit and others show no change. Read the results of conflicting studies in medical articles. If the dosage of vitamins is hotly debated, drug dosages and ethnicity is another topic in the research arena.

Some people have inherited risks for certain chronic diseases. Those people need to eat foods and perhaps take nutritional supplements that will prevent or delay the onset of those problems. Nutritional genomics fills an important need in maintaining health and quality of life. From the *Institute of Food Research (IFR)* in Norwich, UK, **Dr. Ruan Elliot, lead IFR scientist,** sent me this e-letter in response to my questions about what is being researched there. Here's the reply.

Dear Anne:

My main research interests are in using so-called functional genomic techniques to define mechanisms by which diet and specific components of the diet promote human health. These powerful techniques are set to revolutionise the way we approach fundamental nutrition research. On top of this, as you will appreciate, there is also the aspect of inter-individual genetic variation, the impact that this has on health and the potential variations in optimal dietary requirements.

To my mind, these two areas are locked together. We need to properly understand the processes by which components of the diet (nutrients, and micronutrients) work individually and together to keep us healthy so as to be able properly to define optimal nutrition for sub-populations or individuals properly based on their genetics.

You can find descriptions of my work and research interests at the following URLs;
   http://www.ifr.ac.uk/public/FoodInfoSheets/EDPgenomics.html,
   http://bmj.com/cgi/reprint/324/7351/1438.pdf

I hope this is helpful.

Best regards,

Ruan Elliott

For further information, contact the Institute of Food Research, Norwich Research Park, Colney, Norwich NR4 7UA, UK. To view their Web site, phone and fax numbers or email address, on the Internet, go to: http://www.ifr.ac.uk/about/.

My philosophy about genetic testing is to remember a quote by Richard Feynman, Nobel Laureate: "The best way to predict the future is to invent it." Your genes are hard-wired for certain foods, but not all foods make compatible software. Consumers need a guide book to nutritional genomics. You'll hear terms such as gene expression, genetic signatures, risk, intelligent foods, and tailoring the food to your genotype. What it all means is that your body is looking for customized nourishment.

If you really want to take charge of your own health and nutrition, learn all that you can possibly find out about how to apply the results of your DNA testing, genotype testing, metabolic, blood, ancestry, racial percentages testing, and body chemistry or allergy testing to what you eat, the nutraceuticals and supplements you select, your exercise style and lifestyle. Everything starts at the cellular level, even the way your body reacts to stress and exercise with cortisol or with relaxation. Individuals react to certain types of exercise, foods, or perceived stress situations differently.

Some nutrients, foods, herbal compounds or other supplements cause relaxation in some people and panic attacks in others. Then there are allergies to consider. It starts with an expression of your genes in reaction to the environment. Some people get an increase in ocular pressure from sleeping on pillows containing a stuffing to which they are allergic. One sip of caffeine can start a panic reaction in one person and relaxation in another. Your reaction is in your genes. It's about body type, another genetic expression, whether you have inherited genes for anxiety of certain lengths, and the whole interplay and interface of one team of genes with another group in your body. I refer to this interplay of genes as a "rhumba of rattlesnakes" at the molecular level.

You have a part to play in all this, and it isn't always as the passive patient or recipient. You have the *genomer* and the *genomee*…Be the *genomer* for a change—the person in the driver's seat. Take control. Take charge of how to interpret your DNA tests for risk and diet changes or for ancestry and family history or for any other purpose for which you want to test your genome or any region of your genetic profile. To be able to understand how to read and interpret a DNA test and apply it to foods and supplements and to know how the foods will actually effect your genetic expression—that kind of knowledge is power.

The information is publicly available in medical school libraries, on the Internet's scientific databases, and in various journals in the nutrition and genetics fields. Most of these sources are open to the public without you having to be a scientist to learn about how your body responds to food at the cellular level.

Start by joining various online groups, visiting your library, and reading the latest medical and scientific journal articles in the field of nutritional genomics. You can network with patient support groups that use genetic testing. Start your own email list message board for consumers who want to learn and listen in addition to sharing resources of information.

The consumer's role is to compare, review, and find out who is best qualified to work with an individual's genes. How does a consumer discern between snake-oil and reputable companies in this growing field? Who is qualified? Consumers need an explanation in plain language what is healthy to eat, not for the world, but for the individual. So it's up to the consumer to do some research and learn a lot more about nutritional genomics.

Beyond food what does an individual's gene expression require in terms of exercise and lifestyle? It's time to educate your body about nutritional genomics and about DNA and ancestry. What foods should you eat and what nutritional supplements (nutraceuticals) would benefit your health? One way to tell is to test your genetic markers.

Which genetic markers? The entire genome? Or specific SNPs that signal risk of certain chronic diseases? Nutritional genomics should be available to all consumers, not only those with money to pay for expensive testing. Sure, in the future the price of genetic testing will come down, but senior citizens and parents today want to know what they can eat that will agree with them and their families.

Researching the Web under "nutritional genomics" I found a company in the United Kingdom called Sciona. According to Sciona's Web site at: http://www.sciona.com/coresite/index.asp?p=1, Sciona is a venture capital backed company that researches and develops tests for common variations in genes which affect your individual response to medicines, food and the environment.

There are around 40,000 genes in the human genome. Sciona identifies those genes that influence a certain function such as cardiovascular status and tests for these as a set or 'panel'. This information is then used by appropriately qualified practitioners to provide you with health advice.

Testing of specific genes rather than the entire genome usually is done by various companies at this time. In the future, the number of genes tested may increase, or science may find which particular genes interact with other genes to put you at risk if you eat certain foods, or whether your specific genes work together in such a way that you can eat almost anything without developing chronic diseases.

According to Sciona's Web site testing specific genes for certain chronic illnesses is useful in guiding aspects of the treatment of diseases such as heart disease and osteoporosis, which are influenced by your genes, lifestyle and environment. For the consumer, knowing which foods to eat to influence your gene expression is important.

According to Sciona's Web site, Sciona's team of geneticists, molecular biologists, medical doctors and dieticians work with universities and other companies to identify the significant genes underlying a particular effect. The effects of these, and other factors such as your diet, are then analyzed to give you specific advice on courses of action tailored to your own genetic makeup and circumstances.

Filling out questionnaires allow consumers to think in terms of focus sheets. Besides DNA testing, food choices, and consultations with your physician, you need to focus on your habits and think how realistically you answer a questionnaire. Think about from which direction you want to participate in nutritional genomics—marketing, research, science, consumer awareness, forming support groups, media, or other. What are your basic interests and how can you apply them to this field? You can contact Market America, Inc. at 1302 Pleasant Ridge Road, Greensboro, NC 27409. Their Web site is at: http://www.marketamerica.com. Here is an e-letter from Andy Aldridge, Public Relations Director, Market America, Inc.

Dear Anne:

After extensive market surveying and testing, Market America and Cellf, a division of Sciona, have partnered together to offer the Nutri-Physical™ Gene SNP DNA Screening Analysis program. This product allows consumers to submit a sample of their DNA to have it analyzed. Once the analysis is complete, consumers receive a report that outlines possible deficiencies along with lifestyle and diet changes that can be carried out to address possible vulnerabilities. To accompany the DNA analysis, Market America also developed a questionnaire that, when analyzed in conjunction with the Gene SNP product, results in a suggested list of customized vitamins and supplements, available in one formula, if desired by the consumer.

The company's Isotonix® Custom Formula makes choosing the correct nutritional supplementation a simple and efficient process. From a Distributor Custom Web Portal, a customer submits answers to a dietary and lifestyle questionnaire and has the option of purchasing a unique custom formula nutraceutical that specifically addresses their individual needs.

Many companies are talking about NutriGenomics. Through our partnership with Cellf for DNA analysis and Garden State Nutritionals for manufacturing and customization, we are actually doing it.

Regards,

Andy Aldridge
Public Relations Director
Market America, Inc.

*   *   *

Consumers Need to Be Involved in Quality Control

You need a voice in quality control. What the consumer needs to understand are the roles of genes in healthcare, and how the *roles of genes* interact when you take in nutrition. Consumers, corporations, venture capitalists the government, taxpayers, and research institutions invest billions of dollars each year to develop this understanding. One example of a consumer group involved in quality control is when parents group together to form their own DNA bank, recruit people to donate DNA for research, and develop databases and Web sites disseminating information on a particular genetic condition.

Consumers can don few or many hats in nutritional genomics. There are avenues to explore varying from watchdog, marketing, research, public relations, parenting, safety, event planning, publishing, gerontology, videography, genealogy, and healthcare, to broadcasting.

If you do your research, you'll find that venture capitalists who in the last decade invested heavily in the computer industry are now looking to invest in biotechnology. The power of gene technology drums up business and communication also for patent attorneys, journalists, and inventors.

To participate in nutritional genomics in a variety of capacities as a consumer, you can write to the United States Food & Drug Administration (FDA), Department of Agriculture (USDA), and National Institutes of Health (NIH), as well as university laboratories, pharmaceutical manufacturers, and government agencies worldwide. Get involved in the power of genetic technology at some level. The FDA is the agency that's responsible for 80 percent of the United States food supply, according to a July 1st 2003 speech given by the Commissioner, Food and Drug Administration.

In that July 1, 2003 speech before Harvard School of Public Health, Mark B. McClellan, MD, PhD, Commissioner, Food and Drug Administration, said, "All of you—consumer advocates, representatives of the food industry, nutrition scientists, and other food experts—have a collective commitment to the issues we face at FDA that is integral to our ability us fulfill our mission. And your help is needed more than ever. Now more than ever, we all must work together to find better solutions."

It's important to read this speech and to look at materials on the Web at the Harvard School of Public Health. Click on the Harvard School of Public Health's Web site at: http://www.hsph.harvard.edu/now/jul11/conference.html. Read the important facts there and check out the forums. The current headline at the Web site notes that "A July 2003 conference at the Harvard School of Public Health 'spurred' dialogue with the nation's food industry on the subject of "'Changing the American Diet' To Improve Health." Read the materials there and think for yourself about how the food you eat is processed and marketed.

In the speech, you'll find key words such as "consumer advocates" and "collective commitment." Your help indeed is needed to work together as a team, to share, with a purpose of finding better solutions. That's why it's important to listen and learn all you can about the future of nutritional genomics. The consumer's involvement is important. The theme emphasized "collaborating to improve the American diet." Collaborating with consumers also means working to decrease obesity and epidemics of diabetes in children.

You can look at the American diet from the point of view of those who work in DNA testing, from those who work with family history and ancestry research, or from those who work in food packaging and processing. It really hits home when you look from the point of view of the consumer or from marketing and product management. Everybody has to eat.

Chapter Five

Consumer Surveillance and Pet Cloning

Bills have been introduced to various levels of government to prevent pet cloning, but no law has been passed as of the date this book goes to press that would prevent cloning of pet animals. Additionally, human stem cell research also has become a current issue in the news. Cell research has been brought to the attention of various levels of government. Human stem cell research is a hot topic in the news and an important trend in scientific study. Besides being part of trends, current events, and news, stem cell research focuses on how genetic diseases can be treated or prevented with the use of human stem cells. Scientific research will continue for the benefit and ultimate health of humankind, regardless of the debate.

There's another branch of nutritional genomics that instead of only testing your DNA to find out which foods are healthiest for your genes, focuses on *manipulating plant micronutrients* to improve human health. See the article on the Internet, a PDF file on a Web site at: **http://www.ipef.br/melhoramento/ genoma/pdfs/dellapenna99.pdf**.

The volume of imported food is growing each year. Consumers have a field cut out for them—surveillance. As FDA increases its examinations and sampling at borders, consumers can work together to research information about food imports and inspection.

A laboratory can only sample so many products. Consumers can take a role in food security, perhaps looking at industry to identify problems or threats. What the consumer's role entails is better information and collaboration. Everyone needs to keep costs down.

Plant biotechnology of food and feed is another area of consumer interest. If you buy food that comes from overseas, do you ever wonder who oversees the packaging and shipping of those products? Are there really enough inspectors to go around? Consumers worry about the widespread use of sugar in soft drinks. In addition to having your DNA tested, you need to understand how what you eat influences your health at all ages.

Another way consumers can oversee quality control is by forming public interest research groups funded by grant money, private donors, institutions, or the government. You can become a volunteer in nutritional genomics, an ombudsman, a lobbyist, or start your own consumer research interest group.

You can turn a hobby of nutritional genomics or DNA for ancestry and genealogy into a business by affiliating yourself with a university lab which you contract to do testing from your DNA testing clients. There are open doors for consumer involvement depending upon your skills and interests. Nutritional genomics needs public speakers and technical writers to relay to the public what innovations the experts are bringing to healthcare and food systems design.

From running a summer camp for teens interested in nutritional genomics internships or learning experiences to recruiting DNA donors to create a DNA bank or in researching and writing about genomics, there are a variety of doors. Consumers have power in numbers. You can even enter as a venture capitalist with a goal of raising funds even if you have no funds of your own and plenty of determination to learn to ropes.

Don't overlook nutritional genomics for the pet care industry from foods to medicine. Contact the veterinary schools about their research on how foods affect genetic signatures of pets or race horses. Check out the Web site for Research Diets at: http://www.researchdiets.com/.

Research Diets, a New Jersey company since 1984 has formulated more than 6,000 distinct *laboratory* animal diets for research in all areas of biology and related fields at hundreds of pharmaceutical, university, and government laboratories around the world. Nutritional genomics isn't only for humans or laboratory animals. Did you ever think about how your dog or cat could benefit by genetic testing to determine which foods are healthiest?

Talk to your veterinarian to see who is researching how nutraceuticals and better food can help your pet's health, especially when the pet is older. What about nutritional genomics for farm animals or pets? Find out who is doing what kind of nutrition research for better health.

Pet Cloning: Can the Feline Survival Instinct be Genetic?

Look at the article on the Web titled, *"Pet Cloning: Separating Facts from Fluff* (published by the American Anti-Vivisection Society in 2005). It's a PDF file on cat cloning at the Web site: http://www.nopetcloning.org/images/report21605.pdf.

Society is divided between those who favor cloning the genes of pets such as cats, and those against pet cloning. Then there's cloning for medical research and commercial pet cloning. The article also contains the history of commercial pet cloning. The first cloned cat was born in 2001. You'll also see other articles on the Web on pet cloning. Mentioned in the article, *"Pet Cloning: Separating Facts from Fluff,* is the case of a cloned cat sold to a woman in Texas for $50,000. Another cloned cat was sold in 2005.

According to the article, "The pet cloning process uses 'surrogate mothers' in whom embryos are planted." The surrogate mother's health is a huge issue because the animal undergoes numerous invasive surgical procedures to implant and remove the fetuses. Who are the watchdogs over pet cloning, pet genetics research, and the pet food industry?

On page four of the article, copyrighted 2005 by the American Anti-Vivisection Society, you can read on the Web the history of commercial pet cloning. According to the article, pet cloning actually began in 1997 when an Arizona billionaire asked an entrepreneurial friend to help him find a team of scientists to clone his dog, Missy. You can read the entire case history. The billionaire invested in a Sausalito, California firm called Genetic Savings & Clone, Inc. (GSC, Inc.). The article notes that the billionaire helped to fund cat and dog cloning experiments at Texas A&M University.

The first successful cat cloning experiment occurred at Texas A&M in December, 2001 with the birth of a kitten named CC. Genetic Savings & Clone along with veterinary scientists at Texas A&M later parted ways because of differing scientific opinions, according to an article in the Bryan-College Station Eagle titled, *"Cloning Firm Says A&M Made 'Mistake' With Cat,"* by J. LeBas, January 29, 2003.

At the end of the article, you'll see references to numerous other articles cited. Use these references as your bibliography to start reading about and researching the field as an investigative reporter would. Perhaps time is ripe for a documentary video on what advances are being made or what research has been done. It's exciting to learn what's out there in the many applications of genetics. When you've done your reading, then it's time to discuss ethics and your role as a general consumer or 'rookie' in the field of genetics.

Also check out *"About Us Our Team,"* (2004) Genetic Savings & Clone, http://www.savingsandclone.com/about_us/team.html. Accessed 03/19/05. Read the article, *"New Breed of Cat, Clones to Make Debut at Annual Show,"* by J.

Barron, New York Times, October 8, 2004. At the Genetic Savings & Clone, Inc. Web site, you'll see explained, "Genetic Savings & Clone employs some of the best minds available in cellular biology, genetics, micro-engineering, computer science, project management, and other fields relevant to cloning pets. This page profiles a few of our key staff and consulting scientists."

Check out their site and review it if you want to be a consumer watchdog of DNA-driven enterprises. Learn about the company so you can make an objective decision on commercial pet cloning and pet DNA industries. The present CEO is Lou Hawthorne, who helped found Genetic Savings & Clone in 1999. According to GSC's Web site at the time this book has gone to press in 2005, the Web page titled "About Us Our Team" notes that Hawthorne has served as the company's CEO ever since. He has served as Project Coordinator of the Missyplicity Project since it began in July 1997.

Before launching Missyplicity, Hawthorne coordinated large-scale technology and media projects both independently and for various Fortune 500 clients. He worked professionally as a media producer focusing on video, software, CD-ROMs and websites. What's Hawthorne's background? Hawthorne received a BA in English Literature from Princeton University in 1983. According to the GSC Web site, he has "6 years of on-the-job life sciences training from top scientists in various disciplines."

In business, the GSC Web site states that "Hawthorne has years of direct training by Dr. John Sperling, GSC's primary investor and founder of Apollo Group, a $15B company frequently identified as one of the best managed companies in the world." Hawthorne works out of GSC's Sausalito, California offices. As the time this book went to press in March 2005, the GSC Web site reported that "Hawthorne works out of GSC's Sausalito, California offices and resides in nearby Mill Valley."

Who was GSC's primary investor? It was Dr. John Sperling. The GSC Web site names the primary investor as, "Dr. John Sperling, GSC's primary investor and founder of Apollo Group, a $15B company frequently identified as one of the best managed companies in the world." The GSC Web site also notes that "Hawthorne has years of direct training by Dr. John Sperling." If you're interested in this area of research, you can sign up for The Dish newsletter published by GSC.

So as a consumer watchdog in the burgeoning genetics and DNA testing or even cloning environment, are you beginning to find a niche for yourself to begin learning more about what affects and impacts your genes and your pet's? If you'd like to read more, check out the articles on GSC's "In the News" Web site at: http://www.savingsandclone.com/news/in_the_news.html

Don't forget to look at the company's many press releases. You can learn a lot and find valuable contacts in your research to review and recommend or be a consumer watchdog in the genetics industries. A February 16, 2005 press release at GSC's press release site at: http://www.savingsandclone.com/news/releases.html begins, "Genetic Savings & Clone (GSC), the world's only pet cloning company, today announced the launch of DefendPetCloning.org, a web site that responds to a new anti—pet—cloning campaign by the American Anti—Vivisection Society (AAVS). The AAVS claims that pet cloning harms animals, exacerbates pet overpopulation, and misleads grieving pet lovers. DefendPetCloning.org shows that GSC provides benefits to animals, both domestic and endangered, reduces pet overpopulation, and provides a valuable service to consumers."

That's why it's important to get all sides of an issue and study the facts, ethics, and entire picture. Make sure the media you look at sees all sides of the issues and ethics. Research the credible media and think for yourself. As a sample, here are two of the several pointers on the Web site. For example, "GSC's DefendPetCloning.org shows:

- The results GSC has achieved using the new chromatin transfer method of cloning are excellent, which is why GSC guarantees the health of the clones it provides to clients.
- The company safeguards the wellbeing of surrogate mother cats and dogs, and uses animal care protocols that exceed the standard of care established for animal research laboratories."

Check out the news releases at: http://www.savingsandclone.com/news/releases.html. Look at other Web sites. Do your research on all sides of the issue before you make up your mind on pet cloning. At the GSC News-Press Releases site, you'll see a February 14, 2005 article titled, *"Latest Cat Cloning Client Has "Happiest Day of My Life," GSC Cuts Price, Announces New Chief Scientist*

The press release notes, Dan, a 40-something investment counselor, became the second paying client to receive a pet clone when Genetic Savings & Clone officials delivered a kitten to his door on Tuesday, February 8. "Little Gizmo" is a clone of Gizmo, his mixed breed Siamese who died at age 13 in March 2004.

"Valentine's Day is a special day for GSC, because our business is all about the love between people and their exceptional pets," said GSC CEO Lou Hawthorne, who delivered Little Gizmo with Mike Hodnett, the company's VP of Sales & Marketing. "With our second commercial cat clone delivery, we have again duplicated an exceptional pet, and made a certain client very, very happy."

Dan, who requested that his last name be withheld for privacy, was among the first five people to sign up for GSC's cat cloning service, which became available in February 2004 on a limited basis at the price of $50,000. One company client received her cloned kitten in December; the others will receive theirs within the next few months.

"There are no words to describe how happy I am," Dan wrote in an email to Hodnett after spending time with Little Gizmo. Company policy is to counsel clients that because behavior is influenced by environment as well as by genes, clones may not behave exactly as their genetic donors did. Nonetheless, both of the clients who have now received clones say that not only do they look like their predecessors, but their behavior is strikingly similar as well.

"She is exact, exact, exact in all of her mannerisms, habits, traits and personality," Dan wrote of Little Gizmo's similarity to Gizmo. Little Gizmo was born in Austin, Texas, where GSC has done most of its cloning research and development. The company's business headquarters is located in Sausalito, California.

Phil Damiani, PhD, GSC's new Chief Scientific Officer, describes Little Gizmo as yet another example of the excellent results the company is achieving with chromatin transfer (CT), the technology GSC has exclusively licensed for use in pet cloning. CT is a more advanced technology than NT, the method used to produce Dolly and most other clones. Every cat produced by GSC except CC, the world's first cat clone, is the result of the CT process.

"Not only has chromatin transfer helped us produce healthy, normal cats," Dr. Damiani said, "but it has also increased our efficiency, which means we require fewer mothers than we would otherwise." The increased efficiency of the CT process is one reason that GSC today announced a reduced price of $32,000 for their cat cloning service.

Before joining GSC, Dr. Damiani worked at several leading cloning companies, coordinating research on cows, pigs, dogs, cats, and endangered species, including the Gaur, an endangered relative of the ox, which he cloned in 2000. Dr. Damiani also worked in South Africa establishing a gene bank and assisted reproduction laboratory for wild animals, and helped establish the cloning program at the Audubon Nature Institute's Center for Research of Endangered Species (AICRES). Dr. Damiani received his doctorate in Reproductive Physiology from the University of Massachusetts, and has numerous publications, patents and patents pending.

"As an animal lover and dog owner, the welfare of animals is very important to me," Dr. Damiani said. "GSC's excellent standards of animal care, combined with the expertise of its scientists, made joining the company an easy choice for me."

Animal welfare is among the ethical issues the company regularly addresses in public communications. GSC hosted a media briefing on "The Ethics of Pet

Cloning" via teleconference on Wednesday, February 16 at 11 a.m. PST. This was followed immediately by a second media briefing on "The Science of Pet Cloning." Each briefing included a question-and-answer period. Interested journalists were instructed to contact GSC for more information at 888–833–6063.

GSC turned five years old on February 14, 2005, having opened on Valentine's Day, 2000. In addition to commercial cat cloning, GSC is intensively researching dog cloning, and expects to produce the first cloned dog in 2005. Interested parties can learn more on the company web site at www.savingsandclone.com, or by calling 888–833–6063."

For further information, here are some of the articles listed at the GSC news site cited above where you can read the full articles.

Woman pays $50,000 for cloned cat
by Colleen McCain Nelson
Dallas Morning News
December 23, 2004

$50,000 Cloned Kitten Truly Isn't One of a Kind
by Alan Zarembo
Los Angeles Times
December 23, 2004

Local Veterinarian On Waiting List To Clone Beloved Pet
by Jennifer Brice
First Coast News
November 17, 2004

New Breed of Cat: Clones to Make Debut at Annual Show
by James Barron
New York Times
October 8, 2004

Cat Cloning Offered to Pet Owners
by Maryann Mott
National Geographic News
March 25, 2004

Refined Cloning Gets Whisker-Close
by Dan Vergano
USA Today
August 4, 2004

Cloning Fluffy
by Charly Travers
The Motley Fool
January 4, 2005

U.S. Company Says It Clones Copy Cats
by Reuters News Service
CNN
August 6, 2004

Copy Cats
by Lisa Sweetingham
Time Out New York
February 26, 2004

Pet Cloning
by Rebecca Stewart
Fox 61 WTIC—TV
Friday, February 25, 2005

Missyplicity goes commercial
by Leslie Pray
The Scientist
November 27, 2002

The ethics of cloning pets
by Lou Hawthorne, CEO, Genetic Savings & Clone
TechTV
March 4, 2002

Cloning cats and dogs
by Victoria Fung
CBS Marketwatch
March 25, 2002

How Many Lives Now?
by Wes Allison
St. Petersburg Times
Sunday, February 24, 2002

She Is The Cat's Meow in Cloning
Seattle Post—Intelligencer
Friday, February 15, 2002

Copy Cats…and Dogs
by Sharon Cohen
Associated Press
Wednesday, July 18, 2001

Cloning Companies, Researchers Banking on Pet Owners' Love of Fido
by Mary Deibel
Scripps Howard News Service
Friday, July 21, 2000

Max Reincarnated
by Leander Kahney
Wired News
Monday, February 28, 2000

Heavy Petting
by John F. Yarbrough
ABCNEWS.com
Wednesday, February 16, 2000

A Modern Day Noah's Ark
by Lee Dye
Special to ABCNEWS.com
Monday, July 19, 1999

If you knew you could never fail, would you secretly covet healthy, living clones of all the pets who ever served as heroes in various wars? Think about it. Was it some genetic advantage that allowed those loyal pets to survive? As a general consumer, with little or no science background, what would your role be in the genetics industry? Watch dog? Cool cat? Reviewer of companies? Evaluator? Observer? Investigative reporter? Client? Investor? Researcher? Chat room hobbyist in DNA discussion groups?

What's your place in predictive medicine, DNA-driven family history, pet care, nutritional genomics, pharmacogenetics, genetics history, research, commerce, journalism, art, drama, oral history, video production, visual anthropology, or genealogy? While you're still in the mood of thinking about cloned cats and how much they can cost, here are some true stories of famous 'hero' cats of World War Two. I sold the following article that I wrote to *Cats and Kittens* magazine in 2005, and it is included below with permission.

True World War Two Famous Cat Stories

Oscar, the seafaring black cat, should have been named Jonah. Oscar began his 'naval' career as official mascot on the German Battleship, Bismarck during World War Two. Oscar roamed the decks, ate his fish rations, and scratched at his posts as the Bismarck battled the British destroyer, Cossack.

When the Cossack sunk the Bismarck, Oscar floated on flotsam. The admiral saw a cat on a wet wood roof in the middle of the ocean and rescued him. Soon tomcat Oscar became the mascot of the Cossack, living pretty much the same cozy cat life, when it was decided to transfer him to the British aircraft carrier, Ark Royal. The admiralty noticed a black cat "walking the plank" and rescued Oscar once more from the floating flotsam. And for a third time, Oscar became the aircraft carrier's mascot and pet cat.

Along came an enemy warship and destroyed the Ark Royal. Oscar survived again by floating on a wooden plank and looking so irresistible that the admirals couldn't help rescuing him. Oscar survived his second shipwreck and third ship, finally to be taken to Gibraltar to be someone's pet. The sailors kept tab of Oscar's nine lives. In Britain, black cats are said to be lucky, that is, from the cat's point of view.

I found this Associated Press news story when I went to photocopy a newspaper dated November 18, 1941, to see what happened in the world the day I was born. The original article about Oscar appeared in the San Francisco newspaper, the *Call-Bulletin* for that day. The title of the article was "*Oscar Has His 9 Lives, but Loses His 3 Ships.*" The Associated Press article began, "*GIBRALTAR, Nov. 18 (AP)—Oscar, the Nazi-reared black cat who has been the pet of three warships, is safe and sound here, but all three ships are at the bottom of the sea. In fact, Oscar has been a Jonah to two navies.*"

Cat stories dating from World War Two take a lot of research to locate. If you think it took courage to be Oscar, the feline mascot of two navies, meet another cat named Windy, the pet of Wing Commander, Guy Gibson, VC, the dambuster of World War II. Windy accompanied Gibson on dangerous war time missions. Windy flew in planes and knew how to swim. This cat put in "more flying hours than most cats," From (Desmond Morris, *Cat World*, Edbury). See the "Famous Cats" Web site at: http://myhome.ispdr.net.au/~pshaw/famous.html And Famous Cats We All Love at: http://petcaretips.net/famous_cats_tony_tiger.html

Whisky, the tabby cat slept in 'luxury' on the HMS Duke of York as the British battleship sunk the German warship, Scharnhorst during World War II. Cats and other animals served as mascots, mine-sniffers, and pets with the British and Commonwealth forces.

Cat mascot, **Susan** attended the D-Day invasion after making herself at home on a landing craft of the Royal Navy. The South African Rifle Unit kept a lion as mascot. If you want to see photos of these World War II cat mascots, their photos are at the Web site: WW2 Mascots (A Special Presentation from Hahn's 50th AP K-9, West Germany), at: http://community-2.webtv.net/Hahn-50thAP-K9/K9History22/ . The site contains actual photos of a few of the World War II cats and also some dogs and other animals that served with the military forces as mascots and pets on board ships, planes, or in the field.

Simon, the black and white "tuxedo cat" mascot aboard the HMS Amethyst, a British Escort Sloop, was the only cat to ever receive the Dickin VC medal in April 1949, soon after World War II ended. You can view Simon with the medal on his collar in a photo currently on the Hahn Web site mentioned above.

Simon became famous, according to the news story on the Hahn Web site, when the cat was aboard the HMS Amethyst, designed for convoy escort duty during the Second World War. That sloop happened to be in China just as Mao Tse-Tung's forces consolidated their hold on the country.

The sloop slipped and became trapped on the Yangtze River. As the Chinese shelled the ship, Simon found a way to hide from the bullets during the siege when the ship was hit 50 times.

Seventeen humans were killed, with 25 wounded. Simon hid in the wreckage. And no one found him for four days. But call it the luck of nine lives, Simon survived on fat, juicy rats that boarded the trapped ship. Picture this image: trapped cat, trapped ship, trapped rats. But Simon quickly found a solution to the survival problem.

By eating the rats and not the human's food, the cat preserved the dwindling human's food supply as the sailors defended themselves.

According to the article about Simon on the Hahn Web site "The Communist forces then besieged the ship for most of the summer. Despite his wounds, Simon, the cat, continued his duties, hunting rats on the trapped ship, helping to preserve the dwindling food supply, until the incident ended. It should be noted, that Simon was the only cat to ever receive the award."

During World War Two, British cats received their just rewards by having college dormitories open to them. The concept of the college cat continues today. The Library rules and Emergency Procedures at Jesus College, in Cambridge, England states, "Please do not let the college cat into the library." Watchful cats feel at home among the academic courts of Cambridge, England.

The cat usually sleeps on the sofas in the college offices and roams the campus. College cats are popular today as they were 65 years ago at Oxford, Hertford College, Strong College, and Jesus College in Cambridge, England. View articles, news, and photos on contemporary college cats in England on the *Collegiate Way* Web site at: http://collegiateway.org/howto/life/college-cats/

America has **The Library Cat Society** at: http://www.ironfrog.com/libcats/lcs.html. The Library Cat Society, founded in 1987 by Phyllis Lahti encourages the establishment of a cat or cats in a library environment.

Library Cats on the Web

According to their Web site, Iron Frog Productions, an award-winning independent film and video production group, puts library cats on the map. To find cats living in libraries, visit the Iron Frog Productions Web site (http://www.std.com/catalyst/ironfrog/). Designed by Catalyst Learning Systems of Cambridge, Massachusetts, the site features the "Library Cats Map of the United States." Select any state on the map, and view a list of the cats known to reside (or to have formerly resided) in libraries in that state.

Address for further information on Library Cat Society is at:
The **Library Cat Society**
PO Box 274 Moorhead, MN 56560

Predictive Medicine and Genetic Testing for Humans or Pets

Tap the venture capitalist watering holes and open your own nutritional genomics business. Consumers can hire, outsource, or contract fee-for-service with licensed healthcare staff and geneticists specializing in nutritional genomics research. It's not difficult to raise funds. Billions already are invested in the gene technology industry. Sometimes parents of children with genetic conditions are the first to band together to form DNA banks for medical research. Don't overlook agri-nutrition. It's about what vegetables and fruits you eat that in turn impact your genes.

Medical schools and research institutions often seek federal grant money. Someone is investing billions for this research. Find out who are the investors. Who benefits from this knowledge first? Who has access? Is it the consumer who pays for testing, healthcare, nutraceuticals, and selected foods? It's up to the consumer to take a look at quality-control of the entire nutritional genomics arena.

Everyone is concerned about cell degeneration from a lack of critical nutrition. Unless you know how your genes are impacted by various foods and nutraceuticals, how can you can decide what's good or bad for your body other than looking at family history?

The consumer is concerned with how nutritional genomics as an area of research is applied to healthcare with a goal of disease prevention. For the consumer with no science background seeking a beginner's guide book to the power of gene technology, the first step is to realize that genomics has applications for many more areas of exploration than nutrition, healthcare, archaeology, genealogy, oral history, and population genetics.

So should you get screened? With the enormous variety of diet books on the market, healthy-eating advice abounds. How do you know what works to keep your arteries unclogged and your organs nourished for the combination of genes you inherited? People are different, but similar advice often is given to everyone.

What you need is a personalized report, time capsule, scrap book, or profile that has not only your genetic test results, but everything about your lifestyle, stress reactions, exercise. For example, if your body reacts to exercise by secreting way too much cortisol, should you be taking vitamin C? Will the vitamin restore to a healthier state or further damage your organs? If the vitamin is prescribed, what amounts of it will work best with your genetic expression or genotype? How do you find out whether this regimen is good for you or not? It is to these types of questions consumers want answers.

Information on food groups, vitamins, minerals, extracts, and nutraceuticals in an easy-to-understand format and binder are what consumers need. You also have to learn how your DNA test was interpreted. If someone interprets the test for you, how can you apply the test results to eating smarter foods for your genotype or selecting the right dosages of nutraceuticals? You'd have to keep paying for advice on every aspect of your nutrition as another branch of healthcare.

If you know the language of your genes or can learn it yourself, it makes your road to a healthier self clearer. Consumers need access to and knowledge of quality control. Who is performing the tests? What kind of medical supervision is officiating at the marriage of healthcare to nutritional genomics? Who is at the top overseeing the quality control—the consumer? It should be. You pay to fund the research in tax dollars. So form your consumer groups and look into quality control in the field of nutritional genomics, DNA testing, and related businesses that will open to serve the consumer and the licensed heath-care professional.

As the power of gene technology reaches the masses, all types of offerings will find a way to apply DNA test results to what you eat, how you exercise, what you wear, your prescribed medicines, therapies of various kinds, what music will change your physiological responses based on your genotype, and even what career, lifestyle, mate, childbearing plans, or hobby you choose.

DNA samples usually are obtained by rubbing a brush swab on the inside of your cheek, completing a questionnaire, and mailing the brush to a testing laboratory. Sometimes in the case of a rare genetic disease, blood samples are taken, but most DNA testing is done with a cotton or felt swab or mouthwash. After several weeks, your physician would get a report to interpret for you for nutritional genomics. In testing DNA for ancestry, the report would be sent directly to you.

How specifically is the report customized for you? Even tiny differences in your genes influence the way your body metabolizes foods and excretes toxins. These reports look for *variations*. Your feedback consists of dietary information. Some companies assess your present eating habits and foods with your genetic profile. Advice is offered. For example, some tests look at the type of meat you eat, whether your meat and fish are smoked.

The tests look at the types of vegetables. How many cruciferous vegetables do you eat—such as cabbage, cauliflower, Brussels sprouts, and broccoli? How many raw vegetables do you eat? How many sprouted legumes or whole grains not processed into flakes? Did you know that cauliflower is a low-carbohydrate vegetable, but broccoli is higher in carbohydrates? Did the sprouts you ate have bacteria on them that affected you?

This is important if you are insulin resistant or have too much insulin pouring outing each time you eat a high-carbohydrate vegetable. For example, pectin consumption results in an insulin release. What kind of antioxidants do you eat? How much folate are you taking in, and how does that folate impact your arteries—neutral, good, or worse?

What types of whole grains are you eating? Are you eating your whole oat groats or eating foods high on a high-glycemic index that rapidly turn to sugar in your blood and require more insulin to be secreted which can lead to other problems in excessive amounts.

Does your genetic profile reveal a need for a Syndrome X diet or other measures to halt the excessive insulin secretion each time you eat carbohydrates or proteins? What kind of weight problems or control do you have?

How much sugar do you eat? Do you drink liquid candy such as soda pop? How do diet drinks affect your genetic expression compared to sugared drinks? What kind of saturated fats do you eat and how does your body react to that kind of fat? Do you smoke? What damage has smoking caused your body? What kind of exercise do you get?

Walking moderately may be enough for your body, and too much exercise could bring about high cortisol levels—the stress hormone. Does your body react to exercise as stressful or relaxing? What allergies do you have? All these questions need to be compared against your genetic signature. What genes are assessed by the testing company? Do you have a genetic propensity to alcoholism? Which gene predisposes you to alcoholism or drug addiction when you are under stress? Did you inherit the anxiety gene? If so, what is the right career for you? Do you have the genes that predispose you to panic disorder? Find out how many genes are studied and which genes relate to what physical aspects of your health?

Look for a company with excellent quality control. Recommendations should be practical and proven. Your goal is to improve short and long-term health and prevent chronic diseases or at least delay them as long as possible. If the food you are prescribed don't make you feel better, find out why. The tests you take and the food or nutraceuticals prescribed should be scientifically proven in reputable studies. You can check out the studies in medical journal articles. Make sure they were not flawed studies or studies so old that new studies have proven opposite conclusions.

How can you tell for sure what risks you have and what needs your genes have for certain foods or nutraceuticals without testing *all* the genes in the human genome of an individual? If all the genes aren't tested, how can science really know everything there is to know about your individual gene expression? What's important to know now—going with what you have available? When will the research teams be ready to reach out to the average consumer of nutritional products and healthcare? Today there is a divide between what's going on in research and what's available to consumers. That's understandable because the research is still going on.

Without knowledge of all your genetic markers, how can you develop a plan for maximum health through nourishment? Why must this plan be in the hands of a licensed professional instead of an informed, self-taught consumer? If the consumer is armed with knowledge of what the individual's genes reveal and how it relates to certain foods and supplements, the consumer than can take back control and power over his or her own health.

Knowing your genes is only a beginning. How do you apply that knowledge to practical applications as in how certain foods affect your body chemistry and metabolism? If you have a plan A and a plan B, and you know the unexpected can always kick in, can you still have that feeling of a little more control over the way your body treats you? In a world so out of control, consumers of healthcare are looking for a semblance more of control and power over their sense of well-being and mood.

Diet books written for the masses may not work well with your particular gene expression. Science no longer tells you that you have inherited some gene mutations or defects. So your gene expression causes certain chemicals in your body not to work normally. Instead, you are told that you have an individual gene expression requiring you to eat this instead of that.

If you eat this combination of food in the morning, that excessive insulin pouring out each time you eat high carbohydrate vegetables or fruits won't narrow your arteries so quickly. It sounds so positive. It's practical, and tells you specifically what you should eat and when and how the food affects particular organs or metabolic and chemical reactions in your body as a result of consuming a particular food or nutraceutical. At last, there's a positive solution.

You can use intelligent food to override your defective genes that put you at risk and nourish your gene expression by fulfilling your genetic signature's deepest nutritional needs. How fast are the professional dietitians and nutritionists tuning in to nutritional genomics?

The key for the average consumer without degrees in nutrition or genetics is to learn how to look at a printout of your genetic markers and be able to interpret what that means in terms of which foods and nutraceuticals to consume for your health based on what you are at risk or pre-disposed to come down with given the right interplay of environment, lifestyle, food, attitude, and perception of stress.

It's not as hard as you think to find this information in libraries and in online databases. Any subject that takes money away from professionals making a living giving advice in any field is going to require effort to learn. The key is to find sources willing to share information. You bet they are around, and a lot of scientists are willing to share. Some scientists are concerned about their careers and reputations. They should be. Some are cautious about with whom they share information.

On the other hand, some scientists do not share. It may not be the fault of the scientists, though. If you look in the archives of the Los Angeles Times, you'll perhaps find an article dated July 18, 2003 titled, "Whose DNA Is it, Anyway?" Read that article. It's about a person whose mother has Alzheimer's disease and who, according to the article, was "trying to coax Alzheimer's patients and their families to donate DNA" to a university. It's not only about one person because more than ten thousand people donated DNA for the cause.

How about you starting a nutritional genomics DNA bank, new support groups, non-profit organizations, online discussion groups, or Web sites such as "Moms for Genome-Tailored Meals?" Think about how many consumers, not scientists, whose families have a condition or who are interested in a condition arrange events to encourage people to donate DNA to research.

How many consumers go out to assisted living complexes, senior centers, adult education classes, gerontology workshops, nursing homes and churches or family meetings to recruit people who have relatives with a certain condition such as Alzheimer's? How many consumers reach out to the actual Alzheimer's sufferers to recruit people to give DNA to science—to research, often located at or connected to various university laboratories? This is one way consumers get involved in science without necessarily having credentials in science.

All it takes is a deep interest to take action and learn more about the subject. Some research companies are independent, founded by scientists, but work closely with a variety of universities. Consumers are involved every day in science, usually on the end of recruiting people for donating DNA, planning events, fund-raising, writing about in the mass media, encouraging children to take an interest in science, acting as ombudsmen in nursing homes, running consumer awareness classes for seniors or parents, working with genealogy societies for various ethnic groups whose DNA is being studied by scientists for diversity, geography, or genetic diseases, and philanthropy are but a few ways to get involved in scientific research.

According to the article, you have a situation where DNA was used to search for Alzheimer's genes. Science itself has a great mission, to someday find a cure. The DNA is like a pointer. What the consumer is at risk for is that the research will stop. When the research stop for whatever reason, who controls the DNA you've donated? Read the Los Angeles Times article, *"Whose DNA Is It, Anyway?"* Think about your own DNA and thousands of others who have donated for testing. Who controls the DNA archive when the research is halted in mid-stream?

Who owns all the DNA samples—including yours? Who will inherit and use the samples and for what type of research? What if you have a group of family members suffering from a condition that inheritable and you don't know whether you'll get the disease or not?

What if you donate DNA along with others hoping it will point toward a cure, but the project ends? It's like the old question of who owns the living embryos in vitro when the project is over? Almost anyone with a nursing, social work, or other allied healthcare background can open a home-based or other business part time online or fulltime recruiting people for medical trials.

Around the world, people give their DNA for medical research. Why do people donate DNA? It's not always to find their ancestry or ethnic origins, because in many cases, results become statistical and no feedback is given to any individual or even to members of an entire group. What shows up are anonymous statistics in scientific journal articles or books. People often give DNA in the hope that science will find a cure for their or their family member's genetic disorder or inheritable disease.

People donate DNA to see whether a new test will work better for them, such as a test of racial percentages, or in the case of a disease, a test that will reveal risk that could be overcome with certain foods or medicines or even gene therapy. People hope that the medical field has a way of injecting normal genes into a child or person that will take hold and correct a defect in the existing gene expression. Part of gene therapy is about the introduction of new genes that could fix the old genetic problem, and often it works in certain cases.

What consumers can do for themselves is to take part in creating lending libraries for DNA. You need to have lending libraries open not only for scientists, but for the consumer to at least read about research. Of course, scientists who actually work in laboratories with DNA could enjoy the free and open access to the DNA managed by special DNA librarians. It helps research move forward. As a consumer you are a taxpayer.

Do you know your tax dollars are paying the cost of much of this scientific research, especially the research going on at state universities? If you are paying for this research, then the scientists are public servants to you, the consumer. You have the right to this information as much as any scientist, since you are paying the bills for the research.

The problem is that not all scientists freely share DNA all the time hoping some other scientist will find a breakthrough. It reminds me of competing journalists on different papers vying for the news scoop of the day. The DNA is collected and sometimes not shared at all.

The reason is that a scientist's career is at stake. In research, a scientist's reputation and job depends too often upon breakthroughs that help the career. Will sharing lift a scientist's career by his or her bootstraps? Sharing could mean the other guy finds the breakthrough first. Then in walk the patent attorneys. Scientists can file patents on genes.

What if your child is autistic? What scientists will share DNA with other scientists in research on autism or Alzheimer's or any other condition? What's your role as a consumer? It's to create a situation for cooperation. Consumers tend to form patient support groups and to build their own DNA banks. That's only one way of taking consumer action in a positive way to move research forward and point toward solutions and cures for the benefit of the health-care recipient—you, the consumer.

What can you do with nutritional genomics that is in your interest? You can continue to build DNA banks backed by consumers with an interest in nutritional genetics or DNA ancestry, or gene testing for disease markers. Share among yourselves. After all, you are not all scientists, and therefore have no career in science about which to be concerned. I speak as a consumer here rather than as a science communicator.

What you can start as a consumer is a movement to pool DNA samples into a managed library and DNA bank open to all scientists. Consumers could have access to reading about the research and learning to interpret their own DNA and other genetic tests of SNPs, since most consumers don't have access to laboratories to perform research. The time for the consumer's role in moving research forward is here, and consumers must learn all they can about how to interpret the entire human genome.

Your first step would be to make a list of the various institutes that study particular conditions of interest to you or written in your genes as your risk condition. Start with the ones funded by you as a taxpayer. Learn more about what your genes show you. When you talk to scientists, you'll find out how many will or will not share anything from information to DNA. Talk to the scientists. Get on emailing lists where scientists talk among themselves. If it really were true that scientists never share information, there wouldn't be any libraries or databases. Once anything is published and is not classified by the government as secret, it's shared through journals and libraries. The idea is to do the same with the raw material, the DNA through gene banks and DNA libraries as well as databases.

You already know some scientists don't like to share raw materials such as DNA with other scientists. Just ask most biology educators at universities to share their experiences with geneticists with consumers, let alone the media. If you think your DNA is a gift to the public like your donation dollars, think patents. What if you're a consumer who works with donors? What if your dream is to see children with certain diseases tested for little cost?

What if there are battles between scientists and hospitals for patents? What if a hospital takes out a patent on your DNA or those of a bunch of donors you as a consumer recruited from your efforts, support group, or fund-raising events? What if the hospital is awarded the patent and starts to charge fees?

What if that results in some testing programs closing? It happens over and over. What if the costs of developing certain types of DNA or other genetic tests are or remain too high? These are all the questions that consumers want answered by scientists, hospitals, research institutions, universities, and licensed healthcare professionals.

When a consumer so enthusiastic about learning all about genetics, DNA for ancestry, or nutritional genomics put effort into raising money and providing DNA donors, the consumer wants to be sure that what's used for research doesn't always go to pay for patents that result in fees and costs to the consumer or any-one else becoming unaffordable just to create or invent the new genetic tests.

Media has created videos romanticizing "gene hunters" poised on the cutting-edge of a new frontier—inner space. Gene hunting is entertainment. Yet there are little controls or rules—not even a law that requires scientists to share DNA with other scientists. If gene hunting is another Wild West frontier focused on indi-viduality of gene expression, where are the public interest research groups here?

Back in 1975 I was a book author employed in a temporary job full time for ten months writing the consumer manuals and handling all incoming calls to the consumer complaint center of a public interest research group. My job was to write a book that ended up in the Attorney General's office. The book was a con-sumer manual of how to effectively complain.

Today, the consumer needs a guidebook or manual to learn how to effectively organize what should be in the public interest—research. That research could be anything from the frontiers of nutritional genomics to the study of food on a disease or the disease itself. Sometimes research is shared with the public long after everyone else knows about it. If it's archaeology, it's shared quickly. If it's gene research, that's another story. Sometimes patents get in the way, sometimes costs, and sometimes egos.

Databases are open to the public. The bioinformatics profession manages databases of bioscience information stored in computer software. You can get a certificate in bioinformatics at many community colleges or through extended study programs at various colleges and get your foot in the door of bioinformatics through an internship course.

On the other hand, you have scientists, universities, private companies, and research institutions vying for money and/or information being returned to them for their work in giving information to the databases that hold DNA information. It's all about your taxpayer dollars.

As consumers, you pay your taxes to the government. In return, the government takes your tax dollars and dangles that big carrot of federal grant money in front of the institutions employing the gene hunters. And if those scientists refuse to share DNA with other, competing scientists, well, they won't get the federal grant money that's really your tax dollars.

So who's at the root here who should be in control? It's you, the consumer because you supply the government with your tax money that makes up the federal grant money that goes to the many of the places that employ scientists who test DNA for research.

Write to the National Institutes of Health and ask who is sharing what with whom. How are your questions answered? You could get yourself a career as a grants writer and work your way up to become a grants administrator. That's a long career route where you never know whether or not you'll be chosen for the job. The highest you might get is as a serious student of grants administration research. Another route is to ask scientists why sharing DNA could destroy their careers. It's all a matter of who gets to publish first.

In my quest to find people to chat with, a few scientists turned me down not because I don't have a science degree, and not because I don't work for a major newspaper or magazine, but because I'm *the first journalist* to write a book on genomic nutrition before the scientists have had a crack at it. And the book isn't for scientists speaking to other scientists, but a consumer's guide to nutritional genomics and ancestry by DNA testing.

Consumers don't need to be slapped in the face with technical jargon unless the genetics terminology is defined in a glossary. The purpose of this book is to inspire consumers to look into the subject of DNA testing not only for deep ancestry, molecular genealogy, or archaeogenetics, but for tailoring intelligent foods to their genetic signatures.

If the buzz words in the news are nutritional genomics, then now is the time to organize. What do consumers perceive as critical needs in the field of DNA testing? The entire area of DNA testing needs direction, quality control, and applications. Most people taking DNA tests would like to know how to interpret the test results in plain language.

You see dozens of books published on population genetics, archaeogenetics, the peopling of various continents, mitochondrial Eve, ethnic DNA, diseases and DNA, ethnic genetic diversity, food intolerance, allergies, inherited illnesses, aging, and DNA for ancestry. How many general-reader type books are published on smart foods based on genetic signatures and SNPs rather than chemical, blood, or metabolic signatures?

Positioning yourself first matters if you're a scientist who must publish and patent. If you're an educator with an academic institution, positioning yourself first in publishing is crucial to your career, even factoring in getting tenure.

A consumer's world is based on sharing. A scientist's world is based on fear of competition. It should not be that way, but it is. And few will admit it. What competition? There's no scarcity here. There's room for everyone? Then how come so many excellent PhDs in various sciences can't find jobs in their field?

If you want to check this out, talk to recruiters in the sciences and find out how many people are out of work with PhDs in a variety of sciences. Is it age discrimination? Ask the recruiters for their experiences. They will share with you in most cases. Try writing a book on careers in genetics. See what the recruiters have to say to you. Some scientists at some research institutions also will tell you that before they can share DNA, they have to get consent from everyone who donated DNA.

What do you do as a consumer? You don't work alone. Power is in numbers. You organize, get people together and pitch in as a growing group to start your own DNA bank, perhaps consisting of DNA donors. Then you'll have the problem of contacting universities and researchers at a wide variety of places to see whether they are interested.

For the average consumer who doesn't want to take any action, just find out what foods are healthier, the problem is simple. Just research your own genes yourself. All your genes interact as a team. And as all these genes work together, you usually can't point to one gene as being responsible for one action or disease. You can have a defect in one gene that causes a problem or only a risk.

Both consumers and geneticists are interested in finding out what mutation happens in a gene that leads to chronic illness at any age. When a gene oozes really bad protein or the wrong amount of protein—what are the results?

The interaction between the rest of your genes and the chemical and metabolic systems go wild at the cellular level. You get sick. Gene hunters who study the mutations in your genes can study mutations for ancestry or for sickness. Different genes are studied for ancestry, and mutations there have little to do with illness. So where does the consumer go to start? That depends on what you want from your DNA—ancestry, or a prescription for intelligent food?

If you're talking about illness, you start with patient support groups. For ancestry, it's the genealogy groups, ethnic groups, and DNA mailing lists online or start an archaeogenetics club or e-mailing list. You can start your own academic journal. For nutritional genomics, the field is wide open for you to start your own DNA collection banks. Who controls your DNA—you or the research 'industry'? You control your DNA, of course. You control the direction of any research performed on your DNA, and it's time to take DNA by the reigns and direct it—yes, you the consumer. Your tax dollars fund research. So take control of your own DNA.

In the field of nutritional genomics, you, the consumer must take charge of your DNA and begin to build collections in DNA banks where the DNA donors are in control of the direction of the research. Nutritional genomics is not only for parents of children with genetic defects that need the research so urgently. It's also for anyone who wants to know what foods to eat to stay healthier for longer periods of time.

You can start organizing family networks to review and compare the nutritional genomics industry. You can build collections of DNA in your own DNA banks and create databases and DNA libraries. Instead of re-inventing the wheel by duplicating the existing databases, fill the gaps where your efforts are needed and rewarded. Go to a variety of genetics, foods, and DNA-related conferences and let people know you are starting your own nutritional genomics DNA bank and/or intelligent food bank.

The skill you need is not a PhD in genetics, but the desire to persuade people to come together. You need to be a catalyst. If you're one of those unemployed people with science training and are good at public speaking, organizing people, and fund-raising, it could be the career you're waiting for.

If you are a parent with no particular skill other than public speaking and an interest to learn all you can about nutritional genomics from self-education, it's a way to take action. Be prepared to outwit Mr. or Ms. Medical Research Politics just as you have outwitted corporate politics and the games your mother never taught you. If you are lucky enough to be a homemaker, this is the perfect part time career—finding loopholes in medical research politics. It works best if you are not a doctor's wife. Being a doctor's mother is even better for this career. And if you're a patent attorney or work for one, this is another ball game.

The first loophole is to form your own group. Work as a group and put your power in the numbers. Work with scientists in a group also. If you have DNA to donate, give it to a group of scientists that you can organize as a group to work together. There's the problem of individual scientists sharing DNA with one another. If there's no group of scientists, ask them to form a group to work with your group. Organize for nutritional genomics.

Pool the scientists, not the DNA. Otherwise, you'll have a bunch of DNA on your hands and no place to store it. You've got to organize scientists together in a group to work with your organization. First, you need to start an organization. It doesn't take a lot of money. It's about people working together. Consumers aren't afraid of competition. Scientists are afraid of competition because positioning oneself first is the rule of the game if they are to keep their jobs or get ahead.

Consumers are parents, kids, or retirees, not scientists or medical researchers whose careers will be harmed by grouping together to share information or DNA. Most scientists will not share DNA with other scientists. You can go to scientists in other countries and talk to them. See if they will pool and share DNA for research. There's a far better solution. Start your own DNA bank. You organize parents—especially ones with a little money or prestige in their non-science careers. These elite parents have enough smarts to do fund-raising and hire people to collect the DNA to put in your own DNA bank.

Who performs the best fund-raising and organizing? Public relations communicators, public speakers, entertainers, and consumer media are in-your-face, for starters. Don't bother the fact-checking scientists who need to hold their jobs by positioning themselves first in publishing the fruits of their research. Contact public relations and marketing people such as fund-raisers and marketing communications managers.

Hire people not afraid to speak out and not afraid to learn about nutritional genomics. Start a DNA bank, a nutritional genomics resource center made up of many families. Collect a lot of DNA. Ask for private donations. Share your DNA bank's DNA with any scientist. Let the medical schools know about you. Again, you don't need any type of academic degree or credentials to organize a DNA bank. You just need to hire a staff to collect the DNA and make it available to medical schools and any other scientist for research. Who owns the DNA? The donors own the genetic material.

If you want to network with other parents and consumers who have done this, contact people who have organized their own DNA banks, such as the Autism Genetic Resource Exchange. They are on the Web at: http://www.agre.org/.

Talk to the medical schools that use the DNA banks. Read the Los Angeles Times article, "Whose DNA Is It, Anyway?" July 18th 2003. The article also mentions how the Autism Genetic Resource Exchange got started. You can do the same for researching nutritional genomics, a field that got started only back in 2000, and you don't have to have a background in any science to organize people, hire staff, and get started recruiting families to join you in creating your own DNA bank. Do you know how much you are needed by the medical schools?

When you speak to scientists, you may get cooperation, but you'll also come across someone who will tell you to scram because you don't have credentials, or in my case, because I make up stories for a living as a novelist, overlooking 35 of my non-fiction books. Don't let anyone distract your attention from your goal by trying to focus your attention on perceived shortcomings. Anyone who turns you away probably wants first position. True love is about making sure the loved one is positioned first. What nutritional genomics needs is a little tender loving care.

Who do you contact as your first customer? Try the *research-oriented* medical schools. They don't have anywhere near the resources to collect as much DNA as they need. Contact the heads of the molecular genetics departments at the medical schools.

Not everyone interested in nutritional genomics will want to start a DNA bank devoted exclusively to nutritional genomics. There's a place for all levels of participation. You can hire a DNA collector or learn how to collect DNA from people if you're a people-person. You can raise money from donations or ask your state for money. Have each donor sign a statement allowing the DNA to be shared by other research scientists.

Find someone who is associated with a reputable laboratory or with a laboratory in a medical college to store the DNA samples. Talk to biostatistics professionals. The more DNA you collect, the better it is for the numbers crunchers. Not much is learned from only a few DNA samples unless you're comparing Neanderthals to modern humans.

Nutritional genomics as an industry and area of science needs its own support groups. Most diseases have support groups. It's time support groups were formed for preventing or delaying genetic risks some people are pre-disposed to from occurring through learning more about smart foods tailored to individual genetic signatures.

What's your solution? Since scientific research is for the benefit of the consumer of healthcare and nutrition, start by going to other consumers and getting feedback by reviewing, comparing, and polling consumers on their experiences with testing. Are the consumers satisfied? What would they like to see improved? Today's consumers of genetic testing have enough money to spend on tests that help them make decisions about food, health, or ancestry research. You've seen Michael Moore's TV Nation. How about creating a video called Nutritional Genomics Nation? If not a video or a media presentation, how about starting a database and a Web site?

Still feeling a bit out of control? No need to. Just talk to the professionals in the field and make friends. Aside from professional competition that makes some scientists want to position themselves first in publishing and patenting, scientists really are friendly, welcoming people—especially when you are positioned to give them the kind of publicity in the media they want at this time. Nutritional genomics is a buzz word in the media. It's a hot topic this year. Scientists are finding this one-chance shot at getting positioned first in the media by publications of the highest repute.

Librarians at medical school libraries and publishers really like it when you read magazines that would otherwise be read by only a few. I used to spend months reading journals at the UCSD medical library to get ideas for topics that would result in books—either novels or nonfiction how-to series. So you, the consumer, also can learn the important connection between how to read the results of a genetic test and how to apply it to choosing the right food.

Right now, that key is in the hands of licensed healthcare professionals and scientists. It's time the consumer learned how to interpret the results of genetic testing and how to apply the results to a better way of eating. Self-education is the answer. And even if you put your life in your doctor's hands, how do you know whether he or she is qualified to make the connection between your genes and recommended foods or whether those foods will work with your specific gene expression?

Find out what shows up in your relatives and what you may or may not have inherited at the molecular level. A test of your biomarkers will at least give you that handle on your own healthcare, foods, and lifestyle. The point is to educate yourself about your individual genetic signature regarding risk and the implications genetic markers have on your health now and in your own future.

Keep your profile private, and use the information to choose the best possible combinations of foods to help prevent or delay any chronic illness for which you may be at risk. You don't have to give your genetic profile to anybody who could use it against you such as insurance companies and employers. What you can use your profile for is to choose the foods that your body needs. Let your gene expression show you what to eat, how much, and when.

When you look for a diagnostic lab, keep in mind that you want to deal with companies that provide their testing to physicians or similar licensed healthcare providers and not to anyone from the general public. The reason is that you need to know how to interpret these tests and how to apply what you learned.

For example, if genetic testing reveals your at risk for a certain chronic disease, how would you know that unless you can look at the genetic markers, see the risk, and be able to judge which foods and supplements would cut that risk. What I'd like to see in the future is that the consumer would directly be able to get that information from publicly available sources while maintaining privacy.

What I like about the company is that they have a Web site with clinician support where you can educate yourself about what to look out for in your own body so you can at least ask important questions when you see your doctor for testing. And for physicians and clinicians, it's an excellent site to become more informed in specific areas.

The ideal situation would be to see the results of your testing and be told what risks you have. Then you'd be able to buy a book or look up enough medical journal articles. In the future, as a consumer I would like to see more consumer education so that your preventive care wouldn't always have to be solely in the hands of your managing physician.

You need to have more control over what you eat to lessen your disease risks. For you as a consumer to concentrate on focused prevention and treatment tailored to your individual genetic signature, you need knowledge. If knowledge is power, than those with the knowledge you need and don't have leaves you pretty powerless. So you have to educate yourself via books and medical journal articles, the Internet's Web sites and asking questions.

When you see your doctor, often you have only a few minutes to ask questions as doctors are pressed for time. Make a list of questions you want to ask. You might want to compare opinions and answers between alternative health care licensed professionals and your usual primary care physicians or HMO nurse practitioners.

Then check out with medical journal articles and news or even consumer feedback and reviews of what you're seeking. If you don't see enough Web sites that review genetic testing companies or research institutions and if you don't see reviews of biotech companies doing research, start your own Web site to review the many companies springing up.

Compare the nutritional genomics companies that deal with licensed healthcare professionals, and get answers, opinions, reviews, comparisons, feedback, polls, and consumer reports. You have consumer reports on cars, mattresses, and washing machines, why not a consumer report site or publication on genetic profiling for nutrition and health? Start a public interest research group on companies that look at genes or look at disease in various ways. You'll learn a lot from consumers just as teachers learn more from their students than from many of their books. Ask for feedback. It's your genes.

Learn the terminology. Find out how nutraceuticals affect your body before you decide what nutraceuticals to take—vitamins, minerals, antioxidants. What works for people with your risk, may not work with your specific genetic signature.

What foods can you as an individual eat to lessen the risk or delay the onset of the chronic ailment for which you are at risk? I'd like to see the entire genome tested, not only a few SNPs for the major chronic diseases, but all the genes.

Since cracking the human genetic code in its entirety is so new, science may not have the full impact of which genes react with what foods to build a healthier you. Does anybody really know today which genes are responsible for the way your body reacts to certain foods, medicine, or lifestyles?

Science can tell you the specific SNPs for certain chronic, degenerative diseases. Think about it, is that all there is—as far as all the genes responsible for those chronic diseases? What about the rest of your genetic signature? Are there hidden files at the cellular level?

Intelligent foods are attracting the attention of the big, international food design systems firms. Who else is interested in nutritional genomics? Rushing into the buzz about nutritional genomics include patent attorneys, genetics counselors, universities, pharmaceutical manufacturers, and physicians. Nutritional genomics also attracts the interest of naturopaths, the alternative health and health food industry, and merchants of nutraceuticals. Then there are the big, international food systems design companies. Anybody interested in health and healing or food and nutrition is paying attention to research in nutritional genomics. It's time for the consumer to do some research.

What is your stance on nutritional genomics? I visualize peering inside my genes every morning to know how my body responds to carbohydrates. I can feel too much insulin being released, hitting me like a bomb when I used to eat donuts and coffee the first thing in the morning. A few minutes later I was in tremors, caught between the sugar and caffeine. Needless to say, the whole process led to hardening of my arteries and more.

Only when I switched to a diet that calmed my body type, intelligent foods for my biomarkers, did I realize the connection between what I ate, how I exercised, and what changes were happening in my body in the past sixty four-plus years. What I needed was foods tailored to my genotype. My relatives eating processed carbohydrates and trans-fatty acids didn't last very long. As the only survivor, I had to listen to what my body was communicating to me at the molecular level, to be aware. The best way to be aware is to listen to how your genes respond to what you eat.

Genes communicate beyond a chemical and metabolic level of consciousness through the language of biomarkers. They alert you to risk or no risk in a measurable, physiological way. And the language shows up not as words but as risks on genetic tests. Sometimes genes mutate or make mistakes in copying. There also are other reasons for defects in specific genes. Or you may not have any defects.

Your biomarkers evolve over millenniums based on what your ancestors ate and the climate in which they lived for the past ten, twenty, or forty thousand years.

You can do something about risk such as lower your homocysteine levels with nutraceuticals and vitamins if the levels are too high. Look for clues in family history, your own blood tests and physical exams…and most important, your genetic risk profile.

That's why knowledge of healing foods tailored for your specific genetic profile should be your right. There are food and nutrient solutions to most risks that show up on tests. It's better to know how to overcome the obstacle than to remain in the dark about what foods will delay or prevent future or present chronic illness. Information about your genetic profile should always be private.

When should it not be private? What if you have a contagious disease or apply for a commercial pilot's license or drive trucks or busses, trains or boats? Then regular medical exams will reveal the expression of your genes as you age. What is your opinion on privacy? Have you looked at the polls on the subject of nutritional genomics? What do you think about genetic testing for nutrition and nutraceuticals? There are allied fields to explore as a consumer.

Research the publications and articles online or in print on pharmacogenetics and phenomics—the sciences of tailoring your medicine and healthcare to your genetic profile. Explore proteomics (drug discovery). Read about bioinformatics (managing bioscience information and statistics in computer databases and using computer science technologies with genetics research. You work with both computer programming and bioscience information.) The information is either on the Web or in medical and science journals you, the consumer can find on the shelves of university and medical school libraries.

You can purchase a library card and make use of medical and science libraries at universities. As a senior citizen in lifelong learning, I was able to purchase a library card through a retirement-age group at my nearest university. There are medical journals you can read in the library or subscribe to. Take notes. Use the Internet to read medical and scientific journals online. Use the library photocopy machine for articles you want to take home if you aren't online. Do your homework and teach yourself about the wonders that are out there in the burgeoning field of nutritional genomics.

It's true that a little knowledge can do a lot of harm, but what you're interested in is for the consumer to be able to self-educate at least to the level of the media, and to have the same access as the media to see what is evolving in fields that look at disease in new ways and in looking at health and preventive nutrition in new ways.

For example, when I used green tea extract to cure my gum problems, my dentist was happy for me. Right now nutritional genomics has buzz appeal. It's in the news. At the root is change. The way scientists look at your health today is that nutrients play your body like a violin. Your entire system is an orchestra, and you have to listen to the music.

How does an orchestra of musicians play together in sync? An orchestra harmonizes by being interactive. Your body is part a team. And the systems biology that nutritional genomics is all about works interactively. First science looked at the parts, and then the whole person. Now science looks at the orchestra playing together in sync, the systems biology at the genetic level. It all works together, and what you eat may be able to keep the symphony in sync, playing a healthier, more stable rhythm. Nutritional genomics is more about your individual genes that your ethnic group as a whole entity. What if you didn't inherit the gene to digest milk properly?

In the book *Archaeogenetics*, McDonald Research Institute Monographs, 2000, there's an excellent article based on a study of lactase diversity titled, *"Lactase Haplotype Diversity in the Old World,"* (chapter 36) page 305, by Edward J. Hollox, Mark Poulter and Dalls M. Swallow. Science knows that lactase persistence is a genetic trait. It shows up in various frequencies in different populations.

The point is you can't point to genetic markers to distinguish one ethnic group or race from another in order to prescribe a certain dosage of a drug or food because there is diversity in individuals. You have to look at the genes, the genetic profile first to see whether the individual inherited a specific genetic marker.

On the other hand, some members of some races react differently to some drugs and foods, and you can't prescribe for one person based on how the majority of his or her ethnic group or race reacts to the drug or food without seeing the genetic profile to see what the individual inherited. I say before you prescribe a dosage consider how the person's ethnic group reacts to that dosage…but know what genes the individual inherited first. That's at the root of nutritional genetics. Because it's such a hot buzz word in the news, there is lot of discussion about the changes going on.

According to a June 2005 article by Rob Stein, Washington Post, titled, "FDA Approves Heart Drug Directed at Black Patients," the Food and Drug Administration on Thursday, June 23, 2005, approved the controversial drug BiDil to treat heart failure "specifically in African-American patients, marking the first time a medication has been targeted at a specific racial group."

Interestingly, the FDA used the term, "personalized medicine." The whole idea of personalized medicine is to determine how certain drugs can significantly improve the quality of life of patients according to their race or ethnicity. When adjusting or tailoring a dosage measurement or the type of drug used, there also is the question of mixture of race. Another question to consider is whether a drug can help some patients based on their race even if the same drug isn't found to be of help to people of another race or ethnicity. The news angle is to study the varying effects of drugs and drug dosages on different races long after biological distinctions between racial groups have been discredited by scientists.

On the other hand, African-Americans and sub-Saharan Africans will benefit by having safe and effective options for treating certain diseases. The goal is to find out what characteristics identify people who have different reactions to a variety of drugs. Personalized medicine is all about tailoring your treatment to your own genetic signature. The question is whether an individual reacts to a drug based on race, or whether an individual of mixed race responds one way or another based on an individual genetic signature.

As consumers, you also have to look at whether a drug company is motivated by financial gain or extra years of patent protection if a certain drug is approved for a specific racial group. Scientists are becoming mighty particular about the reputation of who they open up to. An old adage that says your own scientific reputation in a relatively new field in the throes of change depends upon not only on who you talk to, with whom you're friends, but also on the reputation of the publication for whom the media person works that you open up to.

That's why it's nearly impossible for a freelance book author who works for no publication and is not under assignment by any editor or publisher to get an interview with a scientist willing to talk about nutritional genomics. I found *almost*, but not all doors closed as far as getting scientists to chat with me online about what's new and what's news in nutritional genomics. Yet, as you see here, some excellent scientists in the field did give me information at no cost to me for my book on their wonderful, new and changing field.

On the other hand, scientists working with DNA testing for ancestry or archaeogenetics, including those in Europe, greeted me warmly. They readily provided comments and quotes freely at no cost to me and with the friendliest of attitudes. So for those scientists who treated me equally well as any other media professional, thank you, I deserved that. I don't write for the tabloids. I don't put down anyone, ever. I write books for the general reader about choices.

Scientists need to protect their careers and reputations, but they also need to remember that the consumer is the bread and butter of the nutritional genomics industry. What the consumer wants most from the nutritional genomics industry besides the profile and the prescribed foods and nutraceuticals are respect and privacy. Grandma knows best here. It's not a matter of preaching to the choir, of scientists selling to physicians, licensed health care professionals, or genetics counselors. The consumer's body as a recipient of healthcare is involved in the product, and the product is more than a genetic profile in a database. The key word is choice.

What's abuzz about nutritional genomics is that one size doesn't fill all ethnic groups when it comes to prescribing dosages of medicine or certain foods based on one's race or country of origin. For example, many people who lived in certain parts of northern or north central Europe for thousands of years mutated a gene to digest milk without symptoms such as gas, bloating, diarrhea, and cramps.

Many people who lived for thousands of years in Southeast Asia did not inherit a mutation to digest milk without symptoms. You can't assume the ethnic group reacts as a whole because there is diversity. Not all Northern Europeans can digest the lactose in milk, and not all Southeast Asians get the runs and gas from drinking milk because of lactase intolerance.

That's why nutritional genomics (nutrigenomics) speaks out in the same way that archaeogenetics by DNA testing speaks about deep ancestry and population expansions. Trends are moving toward eating and treating according to your own genetic signature. Personalized medicine includes phrases such as *"eat 'bright' for your genotype."* It seems to be a word play on a NY Times best-selling book titled *Eat Right 4 Your Type* by Dr. Peter D'Adamo. The Web site is at: http://www.dadamo.com/. There are lists of medical journal articles in the book. You can learn about the scientific basis of how lectins work. Educate yourself about the scientific links between blood types and nutrition. Dr. Peter D'Adamo, is the author of *Eat Right 4 Your Type, Cook Right 4 Your Type*, and the *Complete Blood Type Diet Encyclopedia.*

The popularity of these diets recommended for the various blood types—O, A, AB, and B are backed by medical journal articles of scientific studies referenced. Eating according to your blood type is a theory, but backed by scientific studies. The entire concept of genetically individualized nutrition seems to have evolved starting with blood type. For example, there are scientific studies of how various lectins agglutinate the blood depending on one's blood type. You can see reviews of many diets at the Diet Reviews and Information Web site at: http://www.chasefreedom.com/eatrightforyourtype2.html.

It's as if the sciences of genetics and nutrition had its roots beginning with blood testing regarding how certain foods affect people with certain blood types. Before the entire human genome code was known, scientists used a metabolic and chemical approach to study how one's food intake influenced one's health. Blood was tested, physiological responses, metabolism, glucose, and other tests to measure anything from allergies to whether one had diabetes. Today we have the whole genome at our fingertips. Tests are costly, but the science is here now.

We don't have to wait another ten years to know how our genes react to food, exercise, environment, relationships, stress, or lifestyle. For example, if you look on the Web you may come across something like this: some people who prescribe nutraceuticals based on blood type might suggest that if you have blood type A, and your body is full of cortisol after heavy exercise, change the exercise or take some vitamin C.

Is this medical education or medical advice? It's a thin line. And the person who puts this suggestion on the Web may or may not have an MD. Naturopaths and nutritionists make suggestions on the Web. How should you react? Look for credibility online and fact-check the various Web sites. Look at the medical articles in journals and read reviews of them, looking for articles commenting on flaws in various studies in anything published.

You can ask your own physician when it comes to medical advice. On the other hand, is your physician trained in nutrition or nutritional genomics? Can your personal physician interpret the results of DNA tests for genetic risks or predispositions? Are you more interested in learning about the issues surrounding gender selection of the infant you want to conceive? Will you be referred to another specialist? Would that specialist be a nutritional genomics consultant, a naturopath, a genetics counselor, a nutritionist, a nurse practitioner, a nutraceuticals company, a testing lab, or who? That's why the consumer needs to take control of his own research about healthcare.

Scientists look at proteins in food and allergies, or whether a certain blood type became agglutinated when a certain food was consumed. Back in the era of World War One blood testing was linked to population genetics. Today, research on the entire human genome code has revealed a more comprehensive way of studying health and nutrition through nutritional genomics. Instead of only looking at blood type and the way food affects you—because your blood type is reflected in how every cell in your body reacts to a certain food—science looks at all your genes.

If you're a consumer with no science background, how can you make money in nutritional genomics? You can put up an informational Web site. Compare, review, and evaluate the genetic testing companies that have contact with consumers. You can compare, review, and evaluate the research companies and the university programs.

Basically, you don't need a degree to develop a consumer-oriented information Web site and/or database or an annual book of facts published for consumers. What you can do is compare what's available to consumers in the field of genetic and genome testing. It can include nutrition, ancestry, pharmacogenetics, nutraceuticals, and related sciences such as phenomics.

You can provide services in a variety of categories even with no science background to start with by listing information on companies as a type of consumer report on the nutritional genomics industry, on the DNA testing for ancestry industry, and related health and nutrition or nutraceutical firms. If you have no money, begin by asking the reputable companies you list for funding.

Talk to experts who know which companies are reputable who can be asked to fund your online business. Ask the food industry for funding. Talk to the patent attorneys. If the universities have little money for research and can't help you, talk to those where the universities go for funding. What government agencies do the universities contact for funding their research in nutritional genomics? What large corporations? Which philanthropists? Start with the largest, international food companies and the healthcare industries.

Then work down to the nutrition companies and the people in alternative health care. If you only want to give out information, that's helpful to the consumer. Develop a database. You want the companies to sponsor your efforts. The first step is to write up a plan and keep knocking on doors. Do a bit of fund raising. If nothing happens, create an informational Web site anyway. I did at www.newswriting.net. My purpose was to give information on genetics, broadcast my talks, and promote my books with excerpts and articles.

Yours may be to compare and review companies involved in any aspect of the DNA testing or genomic profiling arena and possibly to review books and publications. You could include feedback from customers of DNA and genome profiling and testing firms, research organizations and institutions, and any company dealing with the public or the healthcare systems and food systems design corporations or the alternative health markets.

Suppose you weren't interested in any business but wanted to check out the reviews and comparisons of DNA testing companies at a Web site. So the possibilities are limited only by your creativity. If someone tells you that you haven't the credentials to do something, start a Web site reviewing and comparing the kind of companies in which you are interested, and let the consumers give you feedback as well as the professionals and experts in that field.

There are two voices to be heard—the consumer's and the expert from the most reputable companies in any field. That's what informational sites are about—selling facts to nontraditional markets, reviewing, and comparing. There's room for more than a few of these informational sites.

Certain people have different responses to nutrition than the majority of people. Twenty percent of people respond one way, twenty percent another way, and sixty percent still another. Do you respond to eating fruits by getting a bulging belly and too much insulin in your blood? Your DNA wants smarter food. Here's the big picture: Your DNA has cultural, biological, and nutritional core identities. Are you ready to look for the smile in your genes? Do mothers know best what foods their children will respond to according to the rules of nutritional genomics? Are the rules in place yet?

Your genes express their biological and cultural components in health or disease based upon the type of foods you eat. Your genes express their needs based on the type of exercise you do to stay fit as well as the way you perceive the stress in your environment. Your DNA is alive. It's conscious. It's a whole you in miniature. I'm a medical journalist interested in finding out my own response to nutrition. So I began by questioning scientists and other experts in genetics.

How about your response to what you eat? It's okay to want to eat smarter by learning to interpret the how-why-when-where-who-what-where of your entire genome and apply it to practical use in eating healing foods and choosing if needed, helpful nutraceuticals. The goal is to get consumers interested in looking at their own picture of health at the molecular level. It's a fantastic subject to learn. Question all authority and think for yourself. Eating for your genotype is here at last to free you from food cravings. Or is it available to all equally—to poor and rich alike? I say it is if you look deep enough into the research available to the public.

If you could get a printout of your entire DNA genome, what would it tell you about smart foods? How far would you go, how much would you pay to stay healthier and to prevent or delay chronic disease? What would you do to preserve your privacy and keep your employer, your HMO, or your primary care physician from looking at your entire genetic profile? The details are in the DNA.

Chapter Six

Who Makes The Rules in Nutritional Genomics?

About what are scientists talking to consumers? Consumers ask for collaboration between scientists in different fields working on similar goals.

From: David Crawford
To: Anne Hart
Sent: Thursday, July 17, 2003 9:00 AM

Dear Anne:

Kudos to you for standing up to the profit warlords, politics and professional jealousy! I am also a "full-time volunteer who writes for the love of science."

Albert Schweitzer said, "A person who is truly happy is the one who has diligently searched and sought out how to serve others". That is our founding truth at Interface Medical Research, Inc.

We work as consultants to the nutragenomic and nutraceutical community. From basic research, product design and development and clinical studies, we are committed to serve the scientific community and public.

We would be tickled to be listed as a service provider in you book. Thank you!

Please use my letter as you see fit.

David S. Crawford, PhD
Research Director
Interface Medical Research, Inc.

545 Farr Avenue
Wadsworth, OH 44281

Thank you, scientists who were willing to talk to me about how foods, genes, and healthcare are linked. It's as if there's a pyramid with your genes at the top and nutrition—foods and nutraceuticals—at one end of the triangle linked to your healthcare at the other angle. It's a triumvirate of intelligent nutrition tailored to your genes.

What I like about the science of bioinformatics is that the field is about managing databases of biological data. The future of bioinformatics helps to ensure that the growing body of information from molecular biology and genome research is placed in the public domain.

Information should be available equally to self-taught freelance writers as well as staff journalists and to the potential consumer of genome testing and research. Information should be accessible freely to all facets of the scientific community in ways that promote scientific progress.

If you need to do some fundraising to establish a DNA bank or support group project, look to celebrities, retired celebrities, media and film producers, and entertainers. Each year movie stars frequently headline Hollywood fundraisers and similar events that bring in money, sometimes in the millions, to donate to causes, most often for various campaign committees or health causes.

You might make some phone calls to see whether celebrities might want to get involved in planning events that would bring people together to raise funds for nutritional genomics-related projects, perhaps on healing foods and individual genomes. You might develop a slogan such as "Don't let your *genome* become your enemy." Think in terms of foods for the majority in the midst of individual genetic differences.

What foods are best for the majority, 60 percent of the population who usually follow food guidelines recommended by healthcare professionals, dieticians and nutritionists based on general physical exams? How do you respond individually to certain foods and diets? Does your immune system go down when you fast or consume sugary foods such as fruit juice, when you exercise or travel? What foods contribute to your well-being?

When you research a study, find out who has done the study and whether it has held up to the critics or was found to be flawed by someone credible. If the study cannot be shown to be flawed, consider it as evidence to explore further. For example, on July 22, 2003, the Bee News Services of the Sacramento Bee, a daily newspaper published an article titled, "Fish Diet May Help Seniors, Study

Says." The sub-title read, "Weekly helpings may cut Alzheimer's risk, doctors argue." The article listed Chicago as the origin of the news article.

What's missing in the article is any mention of what study the news piece referred to. The subject of the news reads: "Older people who eat fish at least once a week may cut their risk of Alzheimer's disease by more than half, a study suggests." The only problem is that the study is not named.

The news article proceeds to mention that the study adds to the evidence that what you eat might influence your risk of developing the chronic illness. What study? It refers to "a growing body of scientific evidence." I would have liked to see the name of the study so I could read the details in a scientific journal that usually publishes abstracts of and articles connected with studies. Where can I find this "body of evidence?"

I want to read the research studies linking various foods to cutting risk of various illnesses for myself. How about you? Is the recommended food good for my genetic expression and everyone else's or only for the twenty percent of the population who can eat most diets and still remain healthy into old age? What about the other twenty percent who can't eat certain foods without damage to their arteries and organs?

What the article does discuss is that the evidence adds to accumulated information on the subject of reducing risk of developing several chronic illnesses such as cancer, Alzheimer's, or heart disease, if people eat a diet rich in fish, fruits, and vegetables and low in saturated fats from red meat.

There are statistics from the Alzheimer's Association in the article. Approximately four million people in the USA are afflicted with Alzheimer's now, and Alzheimer's cases are expected to rise to 14 million by 2050. The evidence presented in the news article was that 'researchers' found "that people 65 and older who had fish once a week had a 60 percent lower risk of Alzheimer's than those who never or rarely ate fish."

Who did the study? Who are the researchers? When was it done? No mention was given of the amount of mercury in the fish eaten. The article mentions that the meals included fish sticks and tuna sandwiches. No mention of whether the tuna was canned, canned with salt or no salt added, canned with oil or water packed, or whether it was fresh tuna or how it was prepared—grilled, fried, or baked, or boiled? Was the research done by the fish industry? What about the warning labels in supermarket's fish departments about the mercury in certain species of fish?

My neighborhood supermarket has a big sign posted at the fish counter for women of child-bearing age or pregnant women to avoid certain types of seafood with the names of the species mentioned due to the mercury levels. I see an article in the August 2003 issue of *Reader's Digest*, a cover story titled, "Hidden

Dangers in Healthy Foods," that connects fish eating with individual reports of nervous system problems, illness, and hair loss due to mercury residues in fish.

Science writers should be accepted as media professionals by the science community without discrimination as to their credentials and should have equal access with all staff media of large newspapers, magazines, or broadcast networks to the growing body of information in genome research or any other area of molecular biology, especially areas related to preventive health and nutrition, foods, and vitamins and minerals.

The bioscience communicator whether self employed or staff employed acts as a go-between, a liaison between the consumer and the healthcare system or research laboratory, a type of educator and ombudsman. The communicator should be respected and allowed to access databases of biological data. Making the complex easier to understand for the consumer is news.

The scientific community should include journalists who specialize in writing about specific areas of science such as genomics without requiring writers to have science degrees. We attend enough genomics seminars, read enough journal articles, observe conventions, and read enough monographs and books to know what questions to ask the experts. In addition to looking toward the media as a liaison and ombudsman, the consumer of genetic testing is concerned about privacy issues.

For nutrition purposes only, results of tests for genetic risks should be private. The whole idea is to lessen the risk before a chronic disease develops. You can change how your genes express themselves based on food and nutraceuticals, but you can't swap your genes for some other genes.

Nutritional genomics is all about effects of intelligent nutrition—smart foods—on how my genes express themselves. Don't laugh at me. Smile. I need to know how specific dietary chemicals will nourish me at the molecular level. You also need to know about the effects of food on your own health.

Your genetic information—a printout of your entire genome—along with a profile interpreting it in terms of risk, disease, and recommendations for foods and/or supplements, should be kept private to be shared only by you and your healthcare professionals, and perhaps your heirs in a time capsule about DNA and medical history to be passed on to future generations.

It's about what makes you tick at the molecular level, about DNA and health, behavior, and mood. If you are what you eat, why should you eat that way, and what will happen to your health at the molecular level when you stray?

Do you metabolize your meal fast or slow—burn your calories quick or over hours? Your genetic profile will give you clues, but you need to learn how to interpret it. And for the time being, you'll find it difficult to learn for yourself and take charge of your healthcare, because getting your entire genome tested is done in reputable places under the supervision of a physician managing your healthcare. You'll have to work hard to take control of your diet and your genes.

You have to work towards taking control of your genetic testing. The only way to do that for now is to learn how to interpret a genetic test of the entire genome and how to apply that to a diet that works for you. You need to get control of your genes. They are yours. The food you eat is yours. Why should putting diet and genes together cost a fortune now and be cheap in a decade? Knowledge is not only power. It saves you a bundle.

Okay, so the doctors need to eat, too. I should know. My son and son-in law are physicians. Just ask their wives about eating smart foods. The point is there are ways to learn how to look at a DNA test and look at a diet and understand how your genes respond to what you eat. Books are online and in the medical libraries. Read them, you autodidactic learners.

Educate yourself. If a social worker can take a two-year masters degree program and become a genetics counselor, and if a nutritionist and a physician can learn to talk to people about what diets are healthiest for them, then you, too can learn to interpret a DNA test of your entire genome.

The trick is finding someone who comes highly recommended to give you your genomic testing. You do need to send your DNA to a lab. Where do you start? Talk to professionals in the field and find out what books and journals they read in order to understand how to interpret the DNA tests. Find out how your genes respond to what you eat. Very few people have the time to be interviewed, but keep asking around.

Find out whether anyone in the field or recently retired will teach an extended studies course for the public. Go to conventions and conferences where professionals in nutritional genomics congregate. Tailor your food and nutrition to your genetic signature.

Have a nutritional genome feast/party. Invite people who can help you match your DNA to your diet or apply for a job in the field. Whatever you do, get a handle on, control of what you eat and how what you eat influences how your genes respond to that food.

Write about your dieting experiences. Go on the radio. Talk to people. Read professional publications. Sign up to receive the news of the industry. Ask yourself whether you want to get into an allied business from another angle where you'd rub elbows with people in the field. However you choose, get your entire genome tested, and find out how your genes respond to recommended diets compared to what you eat now. The whole industry is moving toward this becoming routine in about ten or more years. If you're as old as I, don't wait, start asking questions now, and find out what foods are healthiest for your genotype.

How does what you eat affect the expression of your genes? Nutritional genomics is causing a rhumba of rattlesnakes in the media. The question for consumers is how to research and interpret one's own genetic signature's response to various foods, medicines, nutritional supplements, cosmetics, and lifestyles before spending money on testing a few genetic markers that reveal risk or predisposition. You'd have to ask smart questions such as whether the genetic risk is only 40% and the lifestyle and food 60% of what might possibly happen to you as you age. It would be wonderful if you could carry an electronic "smart card" with your genetic signature showing how you respond to various drugs, anesthesia, foods, cosmetics, vitamins/minerals/fatty acids, and lifestyles.

If you don't know how to interpret your DNA test for nutrition, you'll need to find a physician who works with nutritional genomics professionals in the medical field and has had training in nutritional genomics. For example, if the physician doesn't have a working contract with nutritional genomics professionals from reputable companies, how will the individual interpret a printout of your entire genome in relation to tailoring your foods? How many physicians today are trained in nutrition let alone nutritional genomics, a field that began around the year 2000?

So check out your healthcare professionals and the companies doing the research to make sure what they offer is what you want. Read the medical journals connected with nutritional genomics. You can find them in local university medical school libraries open to the public. Read some of the latest journals in the field. Go to conventions and attend meetings of associations of professionals who are connected with nutritional genomics and ask for reputable referrals. You can network with people in the field. Read about what research is being done by various companies.

Who is watching the watchers? Is there a genteel vigilante in every field with credibility in national media who makes the complex easy to understand in plain language? In the fifties, the DNA helix was big news with Watson and Crick visualizing the double helix. Now it is public information that science has spectrometers, and you can find bioinformatics databases that manage genetic-related information. You can have a genetic profile compared and cross-referenced to your blood chemistry, metabolic tests, or any other areas of your physical exam or genetic profile.

You can look at genetic risks and find the foods and nutraceuticals that will help you. If you know eating fruit all day will make your blood sugar problems worse, because too much insulin is released into your bloodstream due to a genetic situation, you have some more control. That's what it's all about—control. It's you armed with ways to override your genes as much as you can with healing foods and nutraceuticals, if needed.

Don't only get tested and then left on your own on the dance floor. You need some kind of medical supervision so you can learn how your test was interpreted and why those foods were prescribed as well as the effects those foods will have on the expression of your genes. You need to look at yourself at the molecular level. When you've self-educated yourself, you can take more control over what you eat knowing why the food affects you the way it does—at the cellular levels. You'll know why you're salt sensitive or not, and what happens inside your cells when you eat foods that make react the way you do.

Everyone takes nourishment expecting to feel well after eating. Don't let the caricature of yourself hold you back from exploring how you react to dietary chemicals in food. Look at the nuances, the changes in concentration of the nutrients you take in. Look at how the chemicals in foods make you feel. Eat certain foods and take your pulse and blood pressure. What makes your physiological responses healthier?

How long does it take between eating and seeing the results in your health? You need to compare your genotype, that genetic information such as your genome, your DNA, and look at the way you respond to a particular food or meal. That's why a lot of diet books don't consider your individuality at the molecular level. Many stop at the metabolic or chemical level or just look at blood types. That's important too, but so is your entire genome, all your genes and markers and DNA. What nourishment do your genes require for you to become healthier, delay the onset of chronic diseases, and feel well?

Your genes shuffle each generation. They recombine. Food, like DNA moves beyond family history, ancestry, and molecular genealogy. You need to realize the cultural, biological, and nutritional components of your genome in order to eat smarter for your genotype.

Here's how to eat bright for your genotype. The new field, blooming since about 2000 is called nutritional genomics. Nutritional genomics link what you eat to your physician-supervised DNA test of your entire genome and your healthcare. Nutritional genomics is about food plus supplements when needed and any medicine and/or supplements termed nutraceuticals.

Your genes will give out the signals of what whole foods are needed to delay or prevent infirmity. Who is going to test that DNA, and who will teach you to interpret the test when you can no longer afford a supervising physician for healthcare and have to feed yourself on your own on what money or lack of it may come?

You can lobby for nutritional genomics to be available to everyone equally. How about the right to have your genome matched to a healthy diet? Why not match your genome to a diet that works to make you healthier? What's happening in this industry?

Consumer, be alert to what can you do now with your DNA as far as practical applications of DNA testing not only for ancestry or population genetics, but for nutritional genomics or infant gender selection? Scientists use the word 'interface' a lot as do business executives and people with day jobs. In nutritional genomics you have to study how to interface between your diet and your genes. Yes, that's you in there in the middle right between your diet and your genes. Now interface. Take a picture of your gene expression. Now smile. Snap. You've just developed a picture of your gene expression. It's profiled and digitally filed. You now have a picture of how you respond to what you eat. I'll say it again scientifically:

Nutritional genomics researches the interface between what you eat and your genetic processes. Scientists analyze your single nucleotide polymorphisms (SNPs)[*1]. Your gene expression is profiled to get a picture of your response to your nutrition.

Individual nutrition is emphasized in the new field of nutritional genomics where you tailor what you eat, the nutritional supplements you take, and your entire health program of diet and exercise, work and lifestyles according to your own genetic profile—your genome. Forget about diets for large numbers of people.

Maybe those diets fit the sixty percent of us who can eat those things, but what about the twenty percent who need tailored menus according to our genes? Or what about the other twenty percent who can eat almost any food and still not develop the main diseases that could stem from eating the foods not right for our genotype—heart disease, hypertension, asthma, hardened arteries, cancer, loss of memory, and more? And are these degenerative diseases linked to changes in our genes? How do the different ethnic groups react to different foods?

All this research shines under the umbrella of nutritional genomics. This year it's tracing ancestry by looking at DNA test results, and next year the focus will be on nutritional genomics, how to tailor what you eat according to your genetic markers. That's where the focus of my next book is. Most people aren't aware of the research being done at universities or at companies targeting research on nutrition and your DNA.

There are new fields within nutritional genomics such as the study of how people's DNA change according to their diets. There's the study of pharmacodiagnostic drugs, and phenomics, tailoring your medicine, therapy, and healthcare or exercise and lifestyle to your genes.

Books abound on eating right for your chemical, blood type, and metabolic systems. At the molecular level, you'll see books popping up on eating bright for your genotype, smart diets for your genetic markers. One diet book will not fit all. You have books on eating for Syndrome X, for diabetes, and other illnesses that appeal to groups, but what about eating bright for your genotype? Studies compare the immune systems of people from different ethnic groups or geographic areas.

This country faces a diabetes epidemic in children. Sugar is added to health foods such as soy milk or almond milk and other foods or beverages to bring people back by taste, even to 'addict' people to the sugar so they should buy more of the health food product in some cases. Sugar causes inflammation, insulin responses, stress, and damages the brain. Your first step is to research how such inflammation is caused by sugar and what happens as you age to your insulin response and cortisol hormone release.

Some health food products are drenched in sugar or salt so that sugar and/or salt-sensitive seniors can't easily find a decent meat substitute that isn't loaded with salt, sugar, or fat. All this happens—in the midst of a revolution of research focusing on tailoring your food to your DNA to prevent or slow down premature degenerative diseases.

Make sure you're working with a reputable company that arranges to work with a managing physician. Beware of companies that test different aspects of your body to predict what to eat as the testing isn't of the complete genome and may not be done with a managing physician to interpret the results of the tests for prescribing your diet.

Don't waste money on incomplete or inaccurate testing. Watch out for testing companies that offer nutritional consulting based on genetic tests for a variety of complex diet-disease-or diet-health associations as they may not be reputable. Find out who is reputable before you spend any money. If you are testing for single gene defects such as PKU or hypolactasia, these can be tested for and diets arranged based on the test results.

Check out reputable companies that offer tests which are supervised. Some companies research the linkages between genes, diet and health. Don't go to a company that offers unsupervised tests. Learn the difference between a research company looking at how genes, diet, and health are linked, and a genetic testing service company. Beware of the unsupervised test or the company selling snake oil when it comes to finding out how your diet is linked to your genes and your health.

How do you know the difference? Talk to professionals in the research field before you think of any testing, and make sure everything done is supervised by a physician managing your personal healthcare who also is participating in research of how health, diet and genes are linked.

Think about all the Japanese who eat a dairy-filled American diet and land up with diseases not found in Japan when they kept the ethnic diet. What happens when other indigenous people take on a processed-food Western diet high in whatever disagrees with the nutritional expression of their genetic markers? It's a horizontal (processed food diets) expression of a vertical desire (better health).

The remedy is tailoring your nutrition—foods and supplements—to your genotype as well as customizing your type of exercise and other lifestyle events.

Perhaps it's time to tailor our DNA to our multitude of ethnic diets and first find out which one we inherited or which diet works for our genetic expression. For me it's Omega 3 oils and low-carbohydrate vegetables, B complex vitamins, whole grains, and the Syndrome X diet, but how can we know for sure until our entire genome is passed through the test, and for now, the test is still expensive?

So we have to guess, perhaps at the mixture of ethnicities, family members and their lifelong genetic expression of what they ate. Look at what your families ate and what it did to them. Did you inherit any of those gene mutations? How has what you ate influenced your own health? The answer may lie in the SNPs, the genetic markers. Stay tuned for reporting on new research. These sciences include not only 'nutrigenomics,' but also tailored diets and understanding your genotype.

Related sciences that look at genetic variation to customize healthcare strategies include proteomics, metabolomics, bioinformatics, biocomputation, and phenomics. It's all about getting the details and the big picture of your nutritional status, requirements, and genotype. You can eat better according to your genotype without having to wait another ten or twenty years before testing your entire genome is affordable.

Start by observing your body's reaction to the nutritional and exercise environment. It's about personalized nutrition and medicine. Nutrients are not just nutrients. You have macronutrients, micronutrients, and antinutrients. The details come out in gene expression. Nutrients can alter your gene expression without changing your genes.

Look at your metabolism, DNA, and gene expression the way you use your DNA test results to trace your ancestry. The door is open to personalize diets and customize your medical care. Under the umbrella of smarter nutrition, DNA plays a role that treats you as an individual rather than a member of a special group.

If you're an older individual, it's not possible to wait another decade to look for a customized smart diet to eat "bright" for your genotype. You can have your DNA tested now. Only be on the alert and research the company you're working with so you don't get scammed. A DNA test of your mtDNA or Y chromosome for deep ancestry is not enough of a test. Neither is a test of your racial percentages.

You need more clues—metabolic, chemical, and genetic clues. There are plenty of books on how to eat according to your metabolism or chemical clues, but you need more genetic information. What you need is your entire individual genetic makeup. If you can get a company to give your entire genome a pass-through and genetic printout, it could be helpful in preparing customized diets to help prevent and ease chronic disease.

The only obstacle is that you'd need either a professional to prepare the diet by interpreting your DNA test of your entire genome, and not all physicians can look at your genes and prescribe a diet. What you'd need would be a qualified, accredited, and experienced nutritional genomic specialist to consult with you, look at your genetic profile, and prescribe a diet. You'd need someone with enough experience in nutrition and genetics to know what foods would be best for you as a person. No diet fits all people, not even all ethnic groups. It must be individualized.

That's why it's called "intelligent nutrition." Smart menus are customized to your genomic profile. You eat at the molecular level. Eating smart for your genotype is science-driven nutrition. You can write a diet book for a specific individual, who's a member of a specific ethnic group of whom you can't prescribe a one-size-fits-all menu for that person within any group. There's too much individual diversity.

Where do you start? Research is the first step for any smart nutritional genomics consumer. You start by reading and going to conventions of food technologists and nutritional genomics professionals and/or students. Do your own homework. Start with reading about the metabolic diets based on an individual's chemistry. A decade ago, it was eating according to your blood type or metabolic type.

Now it's eating according to your entire genetic profile, your genome. The trend is becoming molecular, eating down to the atomic level in your molecules. That's because your genes express themselves at the molecular level, within and from the cells. The "eat according to your individual profile" movement began with alternative healing movements that always are keyed into scientific research at the genetic, molecular, and chemical/metabolic levels.

In most every alternative and holistic health magazine you find, the footnotes contain references to studies and medical journal articles. Check those out. It's a good use of time to learn how to read articles in medical journals and look up the terminology. If a study is flawed and is reviewed in another publication, read it. If a study holds up with time, keep a scrapbook of the study or articles for your reference.

Only now it's beyond looking at blood type or the lectins that agglutinate your blood from harsh reactions to foods, individual reactions. It's beyond chemical and metabolic, it's now genetic. You inherit and pass on recombination of genes that express themselves in various, individual ways, even within the same family. How you react to food is genetically determined and expressed not only in and through the genes, but also in behavior, mood, and sense of well-being.

Think of the potential for this science-driven food-for-health industry. You must explore the innovations and find professionals to network with to explore and evaluate the forthcoming innovations. Get on the mailing lists of the nutritional genomic research institutions. These research institutions may not do genetic testing of individuals for diets, but are engaged in the type of research you want to learn about before you put your health in the hands of a managing physician who must not only interpret your genome but prescribe diets and/or nutraceuticals.

You've heard of pharmaceuticals. Well, think nutrition and nutrition supplements. Research those nutraceuticals. Make sure everything is supervised, but that you still have an opportunity to learn about why and how your genes respond to what's prescribed, that is, you still have control over what goes into your body and knowledge of how it will affect your health. After you've finished being supervised for your own health, learn all you can about how genes and the diet work together to make you healthier. Then take control of your diet and celebrate your knowledge of a new language—a way to communicate with the expression coming from your genes.

Nutritional genomics is a science dedicated to researching smart diets customized for individuals with a purpose of creating a healthier population. Ask yourself as a consumer, how come it's so expensive right now to test the entire genome of a human to get a prescribed diet and so cheap to test the entire genome of a dog or race horse for breeding or diet? Lobby for costs to come down so diets can be prescribed according to one's genotype.

Besides the research scientists working or studying the field of nutritional genomics in academic or consumer consulting capacities, you have food industry leaders flocking to hear the scientists specializing in genetics and nutrition because the field is potentially a money-making enterprise for nutritional genomics-based food industries.

The whole idea of nutritional genomics got its wings around the year 2000 when studies revealed that a "dumb diet" as opposed to a "smart diet" (based on your gene expression) can fan the flames of your chronic disease risk. So to prevent or delay the chronic diseases for which your genes may be at risk, a diet prescribed only for your genes would help delay or prevent those chronic illnesses. You would need a printout of your genes based on DNA testing to find out for what diseases you may be at risk. Then the diet would be prescribed to prevent or delay those diseases.

Not only the diet, but the exercises and lifestyle and any other nutritional supplements would be recommended. The idea of an intelligent diet would be to nourish your genes at the molecular level based on what the genes needed to express themselves in the healthiest way possible for you as an individual.

So why wait a decade for science to come up with prescriptive diets? There's a lot you can do today with DNA testing and biotechnology before the impact on medical care, on the way foods are processed or not processed, and on your own health becomes influenced by the bottom line—profit.

Science has mapped the human genome. Back in 2001, you have the beginnings of the "marriage" between genomics—mapping your genes, and medicine. You have alternative medicine clawing at the door for decades demanding this knowledge and using it long before the medical fields ever thought of offering courses in nutrition beyond an introduction.

Now medicine and science is working to identify how genes work to change your health. In the meantime, the alternative health books have been emphasizing this all along—how to eat according to your body type, your blood type, your metabolic type, your chemistry, for years. Now medicine and the food industry are finally listening. The turning point came when the functions of various genes were identified with the aim of finding out how these functions affect your health, your risk of disease, and how the genes interplay with your lifestyle, environment, stress level, and even how you spend your day, let alone what you eat.

What you want to know now, especially if you're an older person who can't afford to eat the wrong foods for the next decade, is how and why your genes predispose you to sickness, premature aging, or obesity. While you're out there fighting for organic food, or worried about how genetically engineered crops will make you ill, here's one more concern: think how food is processed and how the process will express itself through your genes. Now customize your diet for your specific needs based on your genes—the expression of your genome based on the foods you eat and the lifestyle and exercise you do. In other words, eat "bright" for your genotype.

What is nutritional genomics? It's a market. It has legal and industrial implications for the food industry. We anthropology and bioscience communicators have been writing about alternative health for decades, exploring the whole oat grains and raw vegetables diets for years, looking at whether fish diets give us lower blood pressure or just a dose of mercury and writing about all sides of the whole foods spectrum, the details and the big picture.

Looking out toward the next decade, nutritional genomics professionals want to attract the baby boomers because of the large size of its population. However, the need is great right now among us parents of baby boomers, the senior silent generation. We are now over sixty and want to reverse our age-related conditions that pop up in the sixties and seventies decade of our lifestyles. We want nutritional genomics now, and we won't wait a decade. So how do we start, our little mtDNA or Y-chromosome DNA tests in hand that we sought to search for our deep maternal or paternal ancestry?

Don't you dare wait for boomers to demand smart diets prescribed for individuals according to their genome. We won't be scammed by diagnostics or counseling aimed at seniors by less than professional firms. We want the nutritional genomics professionals to be our entrepreneurs. To ensure this, we stick to the whole organic foods, but wonder which foods are best to nourish our genetic needs—cooked, or raw? What specific foods are good for us as individuals, and who will prescribe them? How much will it cost? How scientifically verifiable is the information?

Could the genomics revolution actually be the alternative health movement and the whole foods movement joining together? Its purpose would be to look at the molecular expression of specific foods on the body. During the past 30 years, I've been attending holistic health conventions hearing lectures on the benefits of Omega 3 fatty acids, flax seed oils, fish oils, whole grains, low-glycemic diets for hyperinsulinism, syndrome X diets, raw vegetables, juicing with the pulp, the affects of too much fruit on triglycerides, how to flatten big bellies caused by eating sugar in people with hyperinsulinism, enzymes, food supplements, vitamins, and minerals, and what's needed to absorb calcium or magnesium, B-vitamins and TMG to reduce high homocysteine.

All of these are reactions expressed through specific genetic problems. And what I had to do 30 years ago was to take a specific, detailed look at how my body reacted physiologically, and change the food, customizing the food based on how that food influenced my physiology, that is the way my genes expressed themselves and reacted.

It always worked for me. Cut out the sugar, and the insulin-resistant aging belly goes down. Exercise, cut the salt, and the symptoms change. Eat those whole grains that have a lower glycemic level, and the hyperinsulinism subsides until the next meal. Your genes are not my genes. What will work for you? Tailor eating to your own molecular level.

Know all about your genes and how food influences the way they express themselves. It is easy to guess at what the genes needed based on the symptoms and bodily response and also by looking at what the wrong diet did to family members who thrived on a Japanese, vegetarian, or Greek diet and succumbed on a high dairy, sugar, bread, coffee, canned tuna, hamburger, fries, too much yogurt, and chicken diet. The clue was to cut the calorie intake in half, and the disease retracted. So you got a handle on what the genes expressed.

A decade ago, I read books on the metabolic approach. I was a fast burner (metabolic), so I was supposed to look younger and thrived on eating protein and fat in the morning. Sugary cereals caused too much insulin and the shakes in the morning and weakness. Eating fish such as cooked salmon fried in olive oil mixed with egg whites in a patty with no salt, but celery seed, garlic, and onion powder felt healthy for breakfast. Oatmeal was too high glycemic and made me weak and shaky.

By working backwards from the symptoms, I could guess at my genes by what strengthened me after eating and gave me energy. Now I can work backgrounds from the general to the specific, from the effects of food on my feelings to the specific genes that put me at risk for the effects of too much insulin or insulin resist-ance and work backwards and forwards to prescribe myself low-glycemic foods that flatten my tummy and make me feel stronger and full of energy throughout the day.

I attended these holistic health fairs since 1970 when they arose out of the nat-ural foods industry and the alternative medicine movement of naturopaths and nutritionists who were trying to get the medical industry to listen to them. Now they are listening as both sides—the alternative medicine and natural foods industries plug into the nutritional genomics research field from one end, and the medical and food industry from the other end. One group is visionary—looking toward the future. The other is benchmarking, based on what sold successfully in the past.

Prehistoric people ate berries in larger quantities than we eat today, when the berries were in season. Nutritional genomics researches diverse health effects for diverse genes. Flavinoid's effects on inflammation and on the nervous system are being researched. Ask yourself what can you eat that will protect your genes? Did prehistoric peoples have better nutrition then than the standard Western diets encouraged today? Did prehistoric peoples have similar genes to what we have today? Or did the slow-mutating regions of our DNA signal reactions to the change in diet and climate?

From the alternative food and health industries I learned about polyphenols. You find it in green tea, red wine extract, and other vegetable tannins. Anthocyanins are a type of polyphenol. According to Polyphenols Laboratories online at: http://www.polyphenols.com/main.php?PHPSESSID=976bfb699f4 c396cfb032a25fa7877fd, "Anthocyanin is a large water-soluble pigment group found in a large number of fruits, vegetables and flowers."

Anthocyanins are the pigments which give plants their brilliant colors ranging from pink through scarlet, purple and blue. Some pharmaceutical effects of antho-cyanins have been suggested, for example in treatment of cardiovascular diseases and in ophthalmology. The antioxidant potentials of anthocyanins are high."

According to Marilyn Sterling, R.D.'s article in the December 2001 Issue of *Nutrition Science News,* "Eaten in large amounts by primitive humans, antho-cyanins are antioxidant flavonoids that protect many body systems. They have some of the strongest physiological effects of any plant compounds, and they are also things of beauty: anthocyanins provide pigment for pansies, petunias, and plums." (Anthocyanins are a separate class of flavonoids from proanthocyanidins, discussed in *NSN* 2000;5(6):231–4.)

Back in folk medicine of the 12th century, bilberry, a bioflavonoid, was fed to young women to induce menstruation. Bilberry *(Vaccinium myrtillus)* is one of several anthocyanins. British pilots during World War II took Bilberry to improve their night vision. So if your genomic profile calls for anthocyanins, at least you'll know what plant pigments in fruit juices or certain wines or in nutraceuticals such as bilberry extract will be of help.

The genes of the plants, such as the genes in the plant pigments feed your genes. The work goes on at the molecular level. Bilberry was used to treat ulcers. If it's found that bilberry may increase the production of stomach mucus to protect the bacteria that causes ulcers from attacking as bilberry was a traditional treatment for ulcers, then folklore herbal medicines may have come full circle to play a role in genomic profiling. See the Web site at http://www.medpalett.no/index.php?lang=en.

Then there are the procyanidins, found in grape seed extract and other plant extracts. I take grape seed extract in a capsule. I heard about polyphenols and procyanidins from the alternative health market and sometimes on radio shows that most people would call the "woo-woo" industry.

Sometimes you hear about nutritional supplements in mainstream media and sometimes in alternative health media. The benefits of nutritional genomics has made it to mainstream mass media with articles in daily newspapers and the NY Times news magazine.

What you as consumers need to do is to read the guidelines of the National Research Council. They are the group that offer guidelines of recommended dietary allowances (RDA) based on the results research. So with advent of nutritional genomics, research may open doors for those guidelines to shift.

Now biotechnology has joined up with talking business applications. The polyphenols found in berries is being researched to relieve arthritis suffering. For the last three decades the holistic food conventions have been touting the same blueberries, grapes, raspberries, blackberries, cherries, to help relieve the pain of arthritis. Grape seed extract which contain procyanidins have been said to help strengthen capillaries.

Now science finds out that eating compounds such as polyphenols found in dark berries inhibits the expression of a particular gene. You still have the arthritis, but the pain lessens or goes away. Does it work? Try it and see how the expression of your particular gene reacts to polyphenols.

The procyanidins in my grape seed extract and the polyphenols in the berries or green tea I consume daily not only strengthened my capillaries, it got rid of my 'rhoids. Then there's body shapes. In Ayurvedic medicine of ancient India, body shapes are divided into vatta, thin, pitta, athletic/muscular, and kapha, rounded, with a layer of fat under the skin. Vatta is less prone to arthritis and more prone to anxiety.

So just by looking at body shapes you gain a handle on something about the expression of your genes. In the health food stores there are recommended food and teas for vatta, pitta, and kapha types. Just read Deepak Chopra's books, and you'll learn.

The wisdom of the ancients around the world knew something about genetic expression. The body shapes are genetic and react differently to foods. A vatta sipping coffee will sometimes feel anxiety from the caffeine (but enjoy a cup of decaffeinated green tea), whereas a kapha may feel the need for the jolt of coffee or regular tea to the nervous system to get going (not be so underaroused). Even without a DNA test, you can look back at reactions to food from the various body shapes and see what foods hit you like a nerve-shattering bomb of hyperinsulinism after you eat, and what food calms you or makes you more alert.

Before you try anything, read the studies and find out which, if any, are flawed, and which stand up to science. Does it work? Only your individual gene can tell you. It speaks not in words, but in the expression of pain or no pain or in other symptoms of strength and energy or weakness and fatigue or chronic illness symptoms. Will your physician work with you? Who will? What about training physicians in nutrigenetics consulting? Will other professionals fill the gap?

What nutritional genomics needs are companies that will sell food that is good for our body organs. Right now I walk into a health food store and find the healthy alternatives to the milk that makes me sick filled with sugar, rice sweeteners, fructose, corn syrup, or other additions, including salt that makes me sicker than drinking milk. Soy milk marked 'plain' is not plain. It's sweetened. You have to look for unsweetened, and most supermarkets don't carry it because they answer when you ask, "Will it sell if it doesn't taste sweet?"

Why are food companies addicting us to sugar knowing we'll come back and buy more of the product? Can it be because of sugar cravings or sugar addictions and not because we want the healthier, alternative products? You have to make your own choices to leave out the sugar, salt, barley malt, rice flour, or other additives that sell the product by possibly addicting you to the taste rather than selling the healthy alternative point. Consider choosing nutrition according to your genetic signature and metabolic system. This is the basis of personalized medicine linking genes to food. Personalized medicine also links genes to treatments, supplements, and medicines. Genes may also be linked to environments. Personalized medicine is still in its infancy.

A few physicians sometimes also produce and sell vitamins, minerals, or vegetarian food products. Are these products best for your particular genome? Does one size fit the masses or only a percentage of people? Food companies need to join forces with nutritional genomics specialists who need to join with physicians, HMO-employed nutritionists, and other health care professionals as well as with genetics counselors. If the food industry doesn't promote food good for specific parts of the body, the people who produce food supplements and other health and diet tools will step in and plug into the genomics field.

If all would work together, food could be produced to normalize cholesterol. However, there is a need to create foods for those who need special foods such as low-salt, low-sugar, and low-fat foods that don't take out one and put in the other. For example, low-fat foods often contain a lot more sugar and/or salt than regular food products. Again, taste is being sold, not health. Look at soy cheese.

Most of it contains 290 mg. of salt. Regular Swiss cheese often contains only 40 mg of salt. Or look at labels of some fat-free cookies with lots more sugar and salt added than you'd find in those unhealthier cookies full of trans-fatty acids, true, but less salt and sugar. My answer is to bake my own cookies.

I take a cup of oat bran mix it with a half cup of flax seed meal and some cooked whole oat groats, add a few almonds, a handful of millet soaked in carrot juice overnight, and sweeten with fruit juice or a banana. I add two or three egg whites and a quarter cup of lecithin granules and a little soy milk if needed. Then I roll out the cookies and bake until light brown at 350 degrees F.

Before you buy low-fat organic alternative food products, look at the label and see whether the sweeteners added will send your blood sugar up. If you are genetically at risk for diabetes II in your mature years, try making your own alternative milk products. Have you check-out the benefits of low-fat goat milk? Look for unsweetened products when you can find them. Talk to supermarkets and convince them that unsweetened products are not marked 'plain' in many cases, and that they will sell, especially to the senior citizens who often don't know where to look for unsweetened or no salt added products.

Know your genes. The old adage "know thyself" means know how your genes express yourself. There are not enough specialized physicians to go around to all the baby boomers who will be knocking down doors in a decade for healthcare. Don't wait for the boomers. Senior citizens must take nutrition into their own hands and do the research on their genes now, not in a decade.

If you're retired, it's time to make nutritional genomics your main hobby as far as researching the effect of food and exercise on your genes. Nutritional genomics is linked to many other scientific areas of study. It's the most important tool for self identity ahead of personality tests and DNA tests for ancestry.

Ally yourself with others researching all the disciplines and branches of the life sciences. Food industry people need to read up on nutritional genomics. You don't need a special degree to know that food changes the way your genes express themselves. The prescribed appropriate and specific food combinations won't change your genes, but it will allow what genes you have to express themselves in the healthiest way they can. Some people may need to change their food or nutritional supplements based on their gene expression.

You could be taking vitamins and minerals in the wrong amounts or emphasizing the wrong supplements. Find out which ones you need and how much according to your genetic needs. Again, you don't have to wait another ten years until this is available to the masses. Do your research homework.

There are ways to find out what works with your genes. Join organizations that focus on allying people in the life sciences. Join the various life sciences alliances. People in many disciplines need to join together. For example the food industry, genomic scientists, healthcare professionals, journalists in bioscience communications, and the alternative health care markets need to plug into one another's research and resources. What's missing from these alliances? It's the consumer. Take charge of your search for self-identity at the genetic level.

If you don't see a new development and you're a consumer, perhaps you can develop it yourself. You don't need a degree in nutrition to make your own soy milk in a blender if you see the food products on the market are adding too much sugar and salt or barley flour to the milk you see on the shelves. Write to the companies. If nothing happens, make your own nutritious food.

The future of nutritional genomics is based on whether it becomes profitable. If it doesn't become profitable, it won't be shelved. It will move to the holistic health markets and the alternative medical markets. The food industry is quick to move in with its own strategies, but it will always be profit as long as there is profit in healthy food. The mission is to convince the buyers in the supermarkets that people will buy food that isn't loaded with sugar, salt, and flour when the fat is taken out.

Nutritional genomics can plug into the phenomics industry—the science of customizing and tailoring your medicine to your genome. The U.S. diagnostics industry is a $2.3 billion business. You want your genotype? Your key-words in your consumer search for companies are "science-based." Contact science-based companies. Most do research, not individual genetic testing, unless it's for single-gene problems. So do your homework and don't bother the research companies if you want a genetic test. What you want to do is search for a managing physician who works with the reputable, scientific-based companies to look at your entire genome before any diet is prescribed.

You want to talk with people who are supervised under an umbrella and find out what research and testing is being done by whom, why, and how, where and when. Don't get taken in by snake oil-type unsupervised testing. Know the company and get recommendations from scientists and attorneys in the genome research business. Do they work with supervising physicians concerning your healthcare?

You can look at a printout of your genes, your genome and conference with health professionals in consultation with you and your nutritional genomics consultants to find out whether a diet alone will help or whether a 'nutraceutical' supplement, medicine, or drug will help you along with the diet. The first place to convince and check out is your own HMO and your insurance company. Find out whether you'll be reimbursed for the expense of having your DNA tested and for any sessions with genetic counselors. Again, don't wait until this becomes common and genetic counselors are flooded with boomers demanding tailored diets and/or nutraceuticals.

What will happen is either the price of the testing will come down or the number of people demanding it will make the price of health care premiums go up, or testing may or may not be covered by insurance in the future when the demand becomes high. You can help yourself now by forming alliances with genetic counselors and research scientists in nutritional genomics. Or at least read their research and join the message boards in nutritional genomics on the Internet. If you don't ask questions now, the answers later could become expensive or scarce, if the price goes down.

Make business alliances with people in nutritional genomics fields. What you're doing is taking research off the shelves of medical school libraries and bringing science to yourself—as a consumer. Again, you don't need a special degree to research this field for your own use. You can become a collector of published research in the field. Clip articles in the news or save Web-based articles for your scrapbook on this subject. Contact people in the news to answer your questions. Get your DNA tested—the whole genome. It's worth the thousand bucks or so now, even if the price goes down to a hundred later. If you get the right diet, ask yourself would it be worth it to your health?

What you want to find out about yourself are the links between your genes and your health care systems. Personalized medicine includes everything from gender selection of your offspring to your food, medicines, and treatments. If you understand yourself, identify yourself at the genetic, molecular level, you'll think differently about your own health. You'll think differently about the health of your children and grandchildren if you think in terms of nutritional genomics as preventative medicine. It could delay the onset of what your genes predispose you to get. If you're at risk, instead of worrying, the dietary change could delay the onset or prevent it.

Time is on your side when you know how your genes express themselves. It's just the molecular you expressing yourself creatively. And since the body is hardwired to try and heal itself, you could lend a helping hand with the specific diet tailored to your genes. A diet book can't fit a whole population any more than one shoe size will fit a whole group of people.

Think about your health at the molecular, cellular level, at the genetic level. It's all about using your DNA for ancestry in a new way, from genealogy to nutritional genomics. Now you can find out whether your vitamins and minerals or other supplements are actually being absorbed and whether you need most of them. If you do, then you'll know which ones are working and which are not.

Food industries, the agribusiness, genomics research, healthcare, and allied life sciences all are working together. The goal is to bring this to the consumer level now and not in the future. You have industries contributing millions to biotechnology centers. Many of these centers are university-based. It's time to bring the university ivory tower lab to the consumer. Food and drug industries are pouring millions into centers to further research. You have only a few scientists working on projects that bring the fields of genomics, nutrition, and health together.

You need more catalysts like this to bring people together to do more than 'interface.' You need consumer action to 'interact' with the scientists who are working in projects that 'interface' the genomics people with the nutrition researchers and the healthcare professionals and genetics counselors. You need consumer involvement and consumer-based research.

You need bioscience communicators to make the complex easy to understand by the consumer with little or no science background. You need the consumer to take charge of his or her own health, privacy, nutrition, and research. Extended studies courses would help bring the consumer into taking charge by learning what research is being done and comparing his own DNA genome test to various interpretations of the test by different professionals such as his or her physician, genetics counselor, nutritionist, and nutritional genomics scientist.

All these fields need to be brought together under an umbrella accessible to the consumer...not in the future, but now, and with the privacy issues intact for the consumer, and the research open to the public in publications or online to be read by consumers as well as by allied science professionals and the media.

Who will write the regulations? It should be up to the consumer to have privacy in individual genetic tests. Genetic profiles are the business of only the person taking the DNA test to be used for planning a diet or lifestyle change. And unless the tests are totally anonymous as to name and address, collections of genomes would benefit scientists studying ethnic groups, but only if there was total anonymity. Nobody wants to be labeled and have somebody else know the label can't be altered. It's too controlling. Privacy should come first. Privacy should be respected so people numbered not by name and address, but by anonymous numbers or letters would ensure the privacy of large groups of people.

Scientists would be eager to collect large numbers of genomes for databases. Your genes are private. They are your time capsule. Your genome test would be something you'd pass on in a family time capsule scrap book to your heirs or future generations to learn about what your genes expressed, what was in the family, and what may or may not have been inherited by heirs.

Each individual has a different genetic pattern due to recombination. Some genes are inherited, but not all. So a time capsule or book binder with your DNA test may be of interest for medical history to your grandchildren, but how much of this they have inherited wouldn't be known unless they had a test themselves and compared genes. The consumer could take an extension course or read about DNA and learn about what, how, and why, when and where the genes express themselves.

Check out the genetic testing products. Do your research so you won't get scammed by companies that could spring up anytime in the future anywhere and target certain customers such as senior citizens or Boomers. Learn which companies are reputable and check them out by satisfied customers and by the reputations of the people who work there. Make sure the companies have professionally trained and experienced people. Check with the universities and the genomic associations and centers to make sure you are being tested by a company they would use themselves.

Most people have no clue as to how to apply genetics to their personal life. Many fear privacy invasions. Few are told what risks and benefits surround eating bright according to your genotype. As regulations come into focus, ask yourself how to validate the testing. When you are able to validate the test, then you know you've learned enough to get tested. Always ask professionals how they validate the genetic test and learn from their answers. Then check out their answers with research and other opinions from various professionals in the field.

What can you teach yourself about the applications of nutritional genomics testing for your individual health concern? How do you apply the information you've read? How do you validate that information? If a company makes a health claim, find out how to prove it and test it before you pay for testing. Pass the word to parents and children about getting their children tested so genetic profiles will be used to prescribe better diets and exercise programs for children as well as parents. Go into the schools and speak at PTA groups on getting children tested.

With the epidemic of diabetes in children increasing, perhaps a genetic profile might help parents to plan healthier diets, beverages, and snacks for children. It might also help the fare in school cafeterias. The idea is to get the word out at the consumer level as to what research they can do as consumers regarding applications of testing and validation of the tests. Then what follows are the smart diets and diaries of changes in health for all ages. The time for tailored eating and lifestyle changes is now.

By the time we wait for cheaper DNA tests of our whole genome and the chance to apply the test results to a practical menu, in what shape will we be? Ask yourself, should what we eat need medical prescription? Learn for yourself. Powerful knowledge is out there for the public and the media. Take control of your genes, your food, and your nutraceuticals. Your destiny will be in the hands of nutritional genomic scientists until you learn the science of nutritional genomics and research how you are impacted at the molecular level by how and what you eat. Reactions to lifestyle, environment, relationships, and exercise, also are expressed through your genes and your body chemistry.

[*1]SNPs see http://www.ornl.gov/TechResources/Human_Genome/faq/snps.html. SNPs are "DNA sequence variations that occur when a single nucleotide (A,T,C,or G) in the genome sequence is altered." The letters are pronounced as "snips."

Chapter Seven

Tailoring Nutrition to Your Genetic Signature

Research has to be applied to thrive, to interest business. Somebody has to fund genomics research for convergence to bring together and link genomics to food systems design and to healthcare. Will it be the largest international food technology companies that funds nutritional genomics as a research tool for better healthcare?

We go from the general—the body—the specific—the genes, from whole foods to nutraceuticals such as concentrated extracts. You end up healthier and with your medical privacy, a special kind of virginity, intact. You also end up with whole foods tailored to your genes instead of tailored foods for the masses in a one-size fits all planet. Foods need to respect your diversity, including extracts and nutraceuticals. That's why exploring what your genes require for health is an innovation you need to learn.

According to Minneapolis-based Cargill's Web site at http://www.cargill.com/about/index.htm, "Cargill, Incorporated is an international marketer, processor and distributor of agricultural, food, financial and industrial products and services with 97,000 employees in 59 countries. The company provides distinctive customer solutions in supply chain management, food applications, and health and nutrition."

Cargill's media release of July 14th 2003 reports that food and pharmaceutical specialties are part of Cargill's Food System Design (FSD) platform, a group of specialty ingredient businesses that formulate integrated food solutions for customers. Cargill Health & Food Technologies is a leading developer, processor and marketer of science-based, healthy ingredients for food and dietary supplements worldwide. H&FT is part of Cargill's Food System Design initiative in which Cargill businesses work with customers to produce ingredient solutions for affordable, nutritious, convenient and appetizing consumer products. H&FT is a business unit of Cargill, Incorporated.

FSD works closely with its customers to produce innovative products and services that deliver nutritious, convenient and good tasting food. It is a unit of Cargill, Incorporated. The idea of new product concept is the result of extensive consumer research. For example, Cargill announced a new product concept in its July 14th 2003 press release, a flavorful raspberry tea that supports bone health. It's one of the concept products unveiled by Cargill Health & Food Technologies (H&FT) at the Institute of Food Technologists' Annual Meeting and Food Expo in Chicago that ran from July 13th–16th, 2003.

Suppose you had a DNA test of your entire genome for the purposes of nutritional genomics analysis and food prescription as part of a health program of diet, exercise, nutrition, lifestyles changes—the works. Assume you have just been counseled by your managing physician and nutritional genomics counselor that the way your genes expressed themselves required certain types of nutrients.

If a particular food or nutrient taken at a certain or any time is what would make your genes respond in a healthier way, delaying or preventing chronic disease now or later in life, then you might reach for what your individual genes might need. Perhaps it would be the refreshing prototype beverage, aptly named Bone Appetit. It contains AdvantaSoy™ isoflavones, Oliggo-Fiber™ inulin and calcium. Emerging science indicates that soy isoflavones may help maintain healthy bones and that inulin may help boost calcium absorption.

Let your genes speak to you by learning the language of your genes—your DNA. Learn or teach yourself what your genes are saying to you. They are alive. They speak. They are you encased in a molecular universe and make up every part of you. Listen for their message. What do your genes whisper in your ear? Is it a need for a prototype beverage? If so, what nutrients are in the beverage that you need?

Visualize your genes expressing themselves in the language of genomics showing you what they require. Up until now, you had to wait for your genes to communicate by your symptoms, by how you felt. Now listen to your genes by how they think. That's what intelligent nutrition is about, not only eating prescribed smart foods, but listening to your smart genes as well.

What nutritional genomics would do in your case is determine whether for you as an individual with a diet tailored to your genes would need a beverage containing soy isoflavones, inulin, and calcium. First, such a DNA test could help you determine whether your body would react healthier or not so healthy to those products. Let's say, it's just what your individual body needs. That's you.

Someone else may show different needs and different reactions to various products. The point is that the food industries have an open door to participating in the whole nutrition genomics revolution. It's like the Internet, with connecting links from your genes to the nutrients your body needs to operate at maximum efficiency.

See the potential for a lot more convergence here of food industries, healthcare, and genomics stemming from cracking the human genome code a few years ago?

It's like the Internet making instant contact between your genes, your food, your healthcare systems, and the food industry. Convergence also works by going from macronutrition to micronutrition, from the holistic you to you at your molecular level, your cellular level. By making right what's inside your cells, the outer you works better. Food system design and your genes are linked through a burgeoning industry and research arena called nutritional genomics. It starts with you having your DNA tested, not just for ancestry, but the whole genome, for links with the healthcare industry.

Currently you have food system design, the healthcare industry, your genes, and the nutritional genomics research area linked and webbed. Compare genetics to the development of the Internet—the all-encompassing net. The idea is basically convergence. You are now a catalyst, bringing various sciences and industries closer together. Business becomes science and science brings research in a more informed well of knowledge.

According to Cargill's July 14th press release, "The functional beverage segment is one of the most innovative in the industry," said Steve Snyder, Cargill H&FT director of sales & marketing. "Based on our consumer research, we know that successful products in this category will be those that taste great and meet consumer demand for products that positively impact health. Clearly, flavored teas fit well into today's healthy consumer's lifestyle. Our goal in creating Bone Appetit and debuting it during IFT is to spur exciting new product ideas with our partners in the food and beverage industry," he said.

Bone Appetit is made with AdvantaSoy™ Clear isoflavones. Proprietary processing technology results in beverages that retain their traditional flavor, color and consistency. "AdvantaSoy™ Clear isoflavones allow us to meet the challenge of creating new functional beverages that promote health and retain the delicious flavor and aroma which made them popular in the first place," said Snyder.

Cargill H&FT provides proprietary science and technology for food applications, new product development, product prototype development and regulatory support. The International Food Technology (IFT) convention attendees were invited to learn more about these products and partnering with Cargill Health & Food Technologies, when they visited booth #1748 at IFT.

Cargill's H&FT business is part of a larger Cargill initiative called Food System Design. As such, Cargill Health & Food Technologies works in concert with customers to produce ingredient breakthroughs and other food system solutions that result in appetizing, nutritious, and convenient consumer products.

Do you eat lecithin granules? I do. I need that particular nutrient for my health. What about you? The food industry also knows you sprinkle lecithin granules on your food for specific reasons related to your health. In Minneapolis, Minnesota and Stuttgart, Arkansas on July 9, 2003, Cargill and Riceland Foods, Inc., announced their intention to form a strategic alliance to manufacture, market and sell innovative lecithin products to food, pharmaceutical, and technical customers worldwide. Under terms of the agreement, lecithin produced by Riceland at its Arkansas (USA) facility will be marketed and distributed by Cargill. The agreement took effect by Sept. 1, 2003.

According to Cargill's July 9th 2003 press release, Riceland, a farmer-owned cooperative based in Stuttgart, Arkansas, has been a leading manufacturer of deoiled lecithin for 25 years. Riceland supplies high quality powdered and granulated deoiled lecithin products globally. Cargill Lecithin has a global sales organization and modern production facilities in Europe and South America.

"The Riceland alliance establishes Cargill as a lecithin supplier in North America," said Jens Heiser, president of Cargill's lecithin product line. "It also supports our goal of growing the lecithin business globally by serving our customers with premium products and the application properties they desire. Well-known brands like LECIGRAN™, LECIPRIME™ and LECIPERSE™ open up exciting development possibilities and are excellent additions to our existing business."

Cargill is a proven leader in lecithin marketing, logistics and identity preserved supply chain solutions. "This alliance is a major growth initiative for Cargill Lecithin and will foster innovation in the deoiled lecithin market," said R. Creager Simpson, president of Cargill's Food & Pharma Specialties North America, where the lecithin product line resides. "It supports Cargill's ability to provide breakthrough solutions with new, value-added products such as identity-preserved, non-genetically modified deoiled lecithin."

Riceland President and CEO Richard E. Bell said the alliance will allow Riceland to operate its lecithin manufacturing facilities at more efficient rates. "In recent years we've been handicapped by not having a source of conventional (non-GM) crude lecithin for processing. This new arrangement with Cargill helps us fill that gap."

According to the press release, lecithin is derived from soybean processing. In its refined liquid form it is used as a natural emulsifier. The deoiling process results in powdered and granular lecithin. Lecithin is used in a variety of foods as a blending agent, dough stabilizer, egg replacer and instantizing aid. It is also an important ingredient in pharmaceuticals, dietary supplements and cosmetics.

Riceland Foods, Inc., a farmer-owned cooperative headquartered in Stuttgart, Ark., has been a leading manufacturer and supplier of liquid and deoiled lecithin products for 25 years. It also operates soybean processing and vegetable oil refining plants and is the world's largest miller and marketer of rice. Its products are marketed globally under the Riceland and Chef-way labels, private labels, as ingredients and in bulk.

So you see the convergence here, the big, international food industries that design food technology systems are *listening* at food conventions to research done by the companies and universities engaged in research in nutritional genomics. Twenty years ago eating health foods was the butt of jokes. You've heard on mass media TV the clichés about how vegetarians and people who walk into health food stores look sickly. You've seen the look of disgust on some people's faces when invited to a vegetarian restaurant. Often they responded with another cliché, "Oh, you're not going to eat those twigs and sprouts?"

The tide has turned. No one makes fun of people who go into health food stores anymore. No one smirks at vegetarians who eat lunch at soup and salad bars instead of taking power lunches with three martinis, steak, fries, and a sedentary afternoon. Yet for some the soup and salad may not work well, and an hour later they are shaking with excessive insulin. On the other hand, the person eating the fatty steak and potatoes might have clogged arteries. So how you react to a meal is determined by your genes—your entire genome, with all its mutations. Some people can eat any type of meal and stay healthy. It's all in your genes as if your genome is a deck of cards shuffling with each generation, excerpt for your mtDNA and Y-chromosomes that pass on your remote ancestry key.

Even as more young people today demand natural food, those types of stores may also sell red meat because some people eat it. There's the competition in those types of stores. And with diets focusing on animal protein versus vegetable protein, the question remains: Will your genes express themselves in excessive insulin both with the high animal protein and high carbohydrate meals? And if so, what's the solution? The Syndrome X diet was helpful to me. What about you? The answer lies in going deeper, that is to the molecular level and seeing how your own genes react to different food combinations.

You'll hear warnings about avoiding the snake-oil companies popping up in the future or here already, but no one dared name them in print. You'll be told to research reputable companies. You'll find out about research companies and DNA testing companies, and learn the difference. Maybe you'll enroll in university programs of research or study and find internships or careers in nutritional genomics. The door is open, but where are the jobs? You don't always have to approach from a research stance into nutritional genomics careers. There are the patent attorneys.

The search for funding for research is real. Who has the money? In the meantime, know your genes. Are you ready for a preventive health profile not only at the chemical or metabolic level, but at the level of your entire genome? Don't forget your pet's genes, either. What food is best for your dog, cat, or race horse? Have you thought about what laboratories are researching in pet-related nutritional genomics? What genomic innovation is next? Let's take a look at ancestry and DNA.

If you're going to learn about how and what to eat for your genotype—your genetic signature—let's consider your ethnic origins. Food is a cultural component. And genes express themselves through cultural components. Genes have more than a biological signature. There's ancestry, ethnicity, and culture to consider when customizing foods. When the media mentions smart foods or intelligent foods, it's more than a perceived consciousness of your genes and the living food nutrients. What is really implied is tailoring or customizing food as you would configure software to your computer's operating system.

You have to tailor the food, choose the food based on what your genes require to function optimally. Since people are more or less diverse within their ethnic group, they may have inherited or not inherited certain genes that express themselves differently with certain foods. One example is milk/lactase tolerance or intolerance. If thirty-six percent of Southern Europeans can tolerate the lactase in milk and the rest cannot, that's one way ethnicity, genes, and food may interact.

If more Northern Europeans can tolerate the lactase in milk without digestive symptoms because ten thousand years ago a gene mutation in Northern Europe (Finland) allowed the people there and subsequently in most of Northern Europe to drink milk—tolerate the lactase in milk—it's a gene expression. If about sixty-eight percent of North American Ashkenazim and approximately sixty-six percent of Greeks can't tolerate the lactase in milk, it's a genetic signature.

How does your body handle certain foods? Find out what foods to eat from genetic testing and profiling. Tailored foods prescribed or recommended should be based on you as one individual rather than the ethnic group to which you belong. People of any one ethnic group are diverse enough to require individual testing. Let *your own genes* point the direction of your nutrition, exercise, and lifestyle plans, not merely the statistical averages of your ethnic group.

Your donated DNA may end up in statistical tables. Are you getting feedback for healthcare, or only a certificate printing out some of your markers? What practical applications can consumers find from DNA testing for nutritional genomics and also from testing DNA for ancestry? If you want to go beyond looking at DNA for deep ancestry or current DNA matches, what's out there for the consumer interested in human genomics?

*   *   *

Can genetic testing reveal whether your genes need a Paleolithic or Neolithic style of eating? If you're not into "fad diets" what do your genes really need to stay healthy in the way of food or supplements? I recommend the book titled,

Complete Food and Nutrition Guide from the American Dietetic Association John Wiley & Sons, NY 2002 (or later editions).

In addition, you need to compare alternative nutrition books, and as a result of DNA testing, find out what your genes really need for nourishment. It's still too early to tell whether the genetic testing is accurate as disease may be caused by mutations in over a hundred different genes. How do you know which genes to research for what need or ailment?

That's why a broad reading approach covers more territory for the beginner until you get enough feedback to make wise choices. Eating is about choices, and taking prescribed or over-the-counter medicines is about knowing how your genes respond to the chemical or the dosage. In the old days, you'd talk to your allergist.

Now you take a DNA test and look at the molecular/cellular level interactions. What if you have the genes or at least the maternal lineages or mtDNA of the oldest human group that first came to Europe or anywhere else? You're only look-ing at two or three percent of your entire genome, but for deep, ancient, ancestry purposes let's have a look. Genealogy buffs and anthropologists enjoy mapping population genetics, particularly the prehistoric migrations.

Haplogroups and Markers: What's a Recessive Gene?

Sometimes a recessive gene is referred to as a form of a gene called a recessive allele. The recessive allele will not express itself if combined with a dominant allele. The recessive allele is expressed by a lower-case letter. Some traits may be caused by having two recessive alleles.

Markers

How many genetic markers can tell us something for various pairings between groups of people? Markers often are great for telling multiple groups apart. For example, one marker in particular can tell Africans apart from all the other groups, but that marker can't tell Europeans from East Asians. Scientists also will look at male Y chromosomes to study various markers.

Markers are different for various ethnic groups. However, there also is some overlap as peoples become mixed. A geneticist can tell the percentages of various races by looking at the markers, even though we have come to accept there really is no such thing as a particular race because of the diversity between peoples in any one race. However, you can still look at genetic markers to see various ethnic group traits for people who have been separated for thousands of years.

African-European	54 markers
African-East Asian	50 markers

African-Native American	50 markers
European-East Asian	45 markers
European-Native American	41 markers
East Asian-Native American	24 markers

What is a Haplogroup? How is it different from a Haplotype?

Your matrilineal or female ancestors inherit the same mtDNA sequences which form a haplogroup. Look at female lineages starting with your mtDNA haplogroup today. It will be the same haplogroup letter as your common ancestor with the same haplogroup letter that lived 21,000 years ago. You are looking at a connection from a single female ancestor to all your direct female line ancestors today.

The sequences within the haplogroup may be slightly different because of the slow mutation rate of the mtDNA, but the haplogroup will be the same. And in some cases, the sequences will be similar to your ancient ancestors. While in other cases, the mutation rate may have changed your mtDNA just a little over that long span of time.

What's a Haplotype?

Let's look at the female lineages, the mitochondrial DNA clues called mtDNA for short.

Individual mitochondrial DNA called for short, mtDNA sequences, is grouped into haplotypes. A haplotype defines a series of special mutations. The mutations when lumped together are called haplogroups. Each haplogroup contains a set of haplotypes descended from the same one common ancestor. How many haplogroups of mtDNA are there? According to Bryan Syke's book, *The Seven Daughters of Eve,* at least 35 mtDNA haplogroups represented by a letter of the alphabet are listed in one of the illustrated tables. Matrilineal (female ancestral) lineages contain the mitochondria.

You can look at ancient ancestry by tracing the mtDNA lines. Some mtDNA letters belong mostly to Africa, while others belong to East Asia. Some are specific to South West Asia (India) and others are found in central and west Eurasia, which includes Europe and the Middle East. Five different mtDNA haplogroups are found in the New World—the Americas, such as ABCD and X, but the differences between the European and Middle Eastern X and the X among some Native American peoples show that they have been separated for thousands of years.

For example, in the book *Mapping Human History,* by Steve Olson, a rare and unusual haplogroup, X showed up among the Algonquian-speaking Native

Americans living around the Great Lakes. It also is present in small amounts in the Lakota and Sioux. Previously mtDNA haplogroup X had been found in Finland and in Italian, Greek, and Druze (Israel and Lebanon) peoples. Haplogroup X so far has not been found in East Asians. How did it get to the New World?

The Native American X mtDNA differed very much from the European haplogroup X to be separated by only one or two thousand years. It had to have come to the New World tens of thousands of years ago. Scientist Douglas Wallace of the Center for Molecular Medicine at Emory University in Atlanta is one of the world's leading experts on mitochondrial genetics. So when he studied two skeletons that lived in the 1300s in Illinois among the Native Americans of that time, he found the skeletons contained traces of haplogroup X.

How did he know it wasn't from mixture with a European? It was the time divergence between the European and the Native American X haplogroup that gave the answer. The haplogroup X in North America had been there for more than 10,000 years. It wasn't a "modern" European who lived in Illinois in the 14th century.

Again, you might ask, perhaps it was a 'Viking' from Finland since X is found in Finland? The tests showed this type of X differs from the European X by mutations that reveal the X that lived in America really had been there more than 10,000 years. So it could have come more than 10,000 years ago from anywhere—central Asia, Siberia. No X haplogroups are in Siberia today as far as one can tell.

Then again, not everyone has been tested there. However, you have to draw the line somewhere, and the differences between the old world and new world X haplogroup were great as if they had been separated more than 10,000 years. It's easy to imagine someone in north central Asia could have joined up with a group of people such as hunters and traveled with them over the Bering Strait while it was still a land bridge more than 12,000 years ago.

What's a Haplogroup?

A group of related haplotypes make up a haplogroup. Haplogroups are studied especially when referring to mitochondrial DNA and Y-chromosomes. If a set of haplotypes are placed into a tree determined by the minimum number of mutations that separate them, the main branches of that tree are haplogroups. Each haplogroup in theory contains haplotypes that are all descended from a single founding individual.

Haplotypes from other regions of the genome are not studied as much because they may not always group together. Recombination makes ancestor-descendant relationships not as specific to see. You have to look for connections when you study haplotypes.

Examples: The vast majority of Native Americans belong to one of four mtDNA haplogroups: A, B, C, and D, but a few Native Americans also belong to haplogroup X. Haplogroup X is found at a low percentage in Europe, but the differences between the European haplogroup X and the Native American haplogroup X show that they separated more than 10,000 years ago.

It's more likely that someone with haplogroup X mtDNA from Southern Siberia, the Caucasus, or central Asia joined a group of hunters headed north and east more than 12,000 years ago when there was a land bridge over the Bering Strait, and settled in what is now called the North American continent.

* What's an allele?

For lots of definitions of these terms, also see the Web site: library.thinkquest.org/18258/noframes/def-allele.htm. Or See: *www.apnet.com/inscight/08271998/allele1.htm*

An allele is a form of a gene. Alleles are located at the same position (locus) on homologous chromosomes and are separated from each other during meiosis. An allele is what is actually within a region of the chromosome, and is found within a gene. An allele is *any of two or more alternative forms of a gene occupying the same chromosomal locus; such as that which determines flower petal color in peas.*

* What's a Haplogroup?

Definition: A bunch of haplotypes make up a haplogroup. The term is used usually when referring to female lineages and mitochondrial DNA or mtDNA. You might call a form of a gene an allele. An allele is an alternative form of a genetic locus. A single allele for each locus is inherited from each parent (e.g., at a locus for eye color the allele might result in blue or brown eyes).

So when a group of alleles on a single chromosome are linked together and usually inherited as a unit, these genes make up a haplogroup. Haplotypes are particularly stable in <u>mitochondrial DNA</u> and on the Y-chromosome, because they are not subject to recombination.

Analyses of mtDNA and Y-chromosome variation usually focus on the haplotype or <u>haplogroup</u> level, rather than comparing exact base pair sequences. In this case, haplotypes are defined on the basis of particular mutations shared by various individual DNA lineages.

Examples: One study of Finnish Y-chromosome variation found that 40% belonged to one of two different haplotypes, which in turn each belonged to different haplogroups and were probably introduced by different founding populations.

* **Genome.** A person's genome is one set of his (or her) genes. The human genes, which control a cell's structure, operation, and division, are located in the cell's nucleus. The full human genome (estimated at 50,000 to 100,000 genes) is present in every cell-nucleus. Many genes are inactive in cells that have some specialized functions. Many cells are differentiated to perform certain functions only.

* **Genes and Chromosomes.** Genes are composed of segments of DNA. In normal cell-nuclei, the DNA is distributed among 46 chromosomes (23 inherited at conception from a person's dad and 23 from mom). Each chromosome consists of one very long strand of DNA and numerous proteins.

The proteins are needed to manage the long DNA molecule. The longest chromosomes each support thousands of genes. Every time a cell divides, the cell must duplicate the 46 chromosomes. Every cell must distribute one copy of each chromosome to the two new cells. When cells stop dividing, that's the end of them and the organism.

* **The DNA Code.** The DNA of each chromosome is composed of units— "nucleotides" of four different types (A, T, G, C). These nucleotides are linked to each other in linear fashion. The necessary sequence of the four types of nucleotides produces the "code" which first determines the function of each particular gene. Then the sequence identifies the gene's start-point and stop-point along the DNA strand. Finally, the sequence allows specified regulatory functions. The code of the human genome consists of more than a billion nucleotides.

The Mitochondrial DNA (mtDNA). Mitochondria are needed for energy in the cell. The mitochondria are inherited from the mother. When tracing ancient and modern ancestry, geneticists look at female lineages or mtDNA. Your mtDNA is passed from mother to daughter over tens of thousands of years with few changes.

MtDNA mutates slowly during thousands of years of migrations of people across the globe. Men inherit their mtDNA from their mothers, but pass on their Y chromosomes to their sons. Women pass their mtDNA to their daughters. On very rare occasions, a few women may inherit some mtDNA from their fathers, but almost all women inherit their mtDNA from their mothers.

What mtDNA Does Not Do: It is not junk DNA. Often DNA produces more copies than it needs to function. Sometimes this is called junk DNA. MtDNA is necessary for providing energy to the cell. Outside the nucleus, human cells also have some "foreign" DNA located in structures called the mitochondria. This small and separate set of DNA does not participate in the 46 human chromosomes.

The mitochondrial DNA (mtDNA) really is not part of "the genomic DNA." According to the "out of Africa" theory that's widely held in acceptance by most scientists, all the mtDNA in the world today came from a single woman called Mitochondrial Eve who had two daughters who survived to create a line of females that expanded all over the world. Similar histories are noted for the male line using the Y chromosome. According to the book, *Mapping Human History*, by Steve Olson, (page 56) "All non-Africans descend from Africans who left the continent within the past 100,000 years."

According to a number of the latest videos on whether people took the northern or southern route out of Africa, the southern route is most favored. According to the book, *Archaeogenetics*, the flow of people varied between then and now. Today, most scientists theorize that since the north route out of Africa most likely was blocked by an Ice Age that created a dry desert in the Middle East, those leaving Africa headed toward Yemen and then along a southern route to India, Malaysia, and finally Australia.

Only when the climate changed and the Fertile Crescent of the Middle East opened up, did people expand back from India toward where the rivers met, the Middle East, such as what today are Iraq and Iran, and the Levant, reaching the coast, and from there north to what today is Europe. About 21,000 years ago, a new Ice Age began, and people who moved up from the Middle East into Europe found refuge in only a few places such as Southwest France, Northern Spain facing the Mediterranean and the Pyrenees, the Balkans and Ukraine, until the last Ice Age ended about 12,500 years ago. Then populations expanded across Europe from Spain to the Urals.

By that time, the Far East had been populated for a long time, and Central Asia was the newest land to be seen. Then by 9,000 years ago, farmers from the Levant and Anatolia moved into Europe and introduced the idea of farming so that about 80 percent of Europeans today consist of the old Paleolithic hunters and about 20 to 26 percent from the more recent arrivals from the Middle East, the cereal belt grain farmers of the Neolithic era that started about 10,000 years ago in the Levant and Fertile Crescent of the Middle East.

Genealogy, history, folklore, oral history, memoirs writing, diary journaling, demography, anthropology, and archaeology are in the midst of a molecular revolution. Has archaeology become archaeogenetics? Actually, molecular genetics biotechnology is one more *tool* in the hands of the genealogist, historian, archaeologist, folklorist, prosopographer, onomasticist, demographer, videographer, anthropologist, or family historian. And that tool, molecular genetics, is used to untangle distantly ancestral as well as recent family roots.

Now you have computer technology and Web databases to research family ties. You have molecular genetics biotechnology—DNA testing, bioinformatics, and beyond.

From ancestry by DNA to racial percentages by markers and phenomics, experts can customize medicine or therapy to an individual's genes.

You can take a paternity test. Or find out whether you're related to a distant cousin you never met. Or you can study DNA as legal evidence. Your genes are used for matching bone marrow donors to recipients. The molecular revolution is enhancing research. From community colleges where students earn one or two-year certificates in biotechnology to perform DNA testing and bioinformatics processing on computers to the PhDs who work in research labs and universities, the molecular revolution has now joined science to history. How much do you want to know about your genome?

*   *   *

Once you found your DNA trail—mtDNA for women, Y-chromosomes for men, and even if you took a racial percentages DNA test, what do you do with the information? You create a time capsule, a scrap book, a type of DNA and oral history journal. You use photography, text, sound, music, speech, video, and you put your ancestral record archive in an oral history—transcribed and put to audio or video, to sound, text and imagery.

You even may want to put your information on the Web or in an archive to be viewed by future descendants. The whole tapestry links you back to that first ancestor and to the one in the future. It's a rich experience in history and time.

How do you write, tape, and transcribe an oral history of your DNA along with your genealogy and family history records and photos? Assuming you're a beginner in genealogy with no science background and interested in family history, where do you begin your search? What's the cultural component behind a trait as biological as your genes?

If you're a family historian, an oral history researcher, or a person fascinated with ancestry, here's how to understand the results of DNA tests. Different people have different, sometimes opposite opinions on whether DNA testing is a useful tool in the hands of family historians. If you are a carrier of a genetic disorder, DNA testing is useful in researching your family history to find out who was the first carrier in your ancestry back in time.

Here the debate unfolds as scientists, authors, physicians, media people, owners of DNA testing companies, genealogists, historians and researchers comment, write, and opine on DNA testing and genealogy.

What is the distribution of mtDNA haplogroup K? We know that haplogroup K is a clade of haplogroup U. Previous studies revealed that 27% to 32% of Ashkenazim have haplogroup K and that 9.0 of Ashkenazim have the mtDNA haplogroup H that follows the CRS. The rest have mutations of haplogroup H that does not follow the sequences of the CRS without mutations. What is the distribution of mtDNA haplogroup K in the rest of the populations sampled?

Take for example one sample appearing in the chapter, *Anatolian and Trans-Caucasus Populations*, Archaeogenetics: DNA and the Population Prehistory of Europe, McDonald Institute Monographs, 2002, page 223. The highest figure is 31.7% in Georgians sampled have haplogroup K mtDNA. Next are Armenians sampled with 27.8% haplogroup K mtDNA. Following are Turks with 24.7%, and Siena, Italy samples, Tuscans, Sardinians, French, and Albanian samples with 35.8% haplogroup K mtDNA. Haplogroup K mtDNA also appears at 25% in the Nile Valley, and at 20% in Ethiopians, and 1.2% of Indians. It also appears at 11% in Estonians, Finns, and Karelians, and at 18.6% in Russians, Poles, Czechs, and Slovaks.

Where did it originate? In the Middle East, probably, but about 17,000 years ago it developed in Europe in the area where Venice, Italy is today and then migrated into the Alps.

How do you use DNA testing to interpret family history records? How eager are people to take a DNA test for family history research? Most DNA tests require only that someone swish mouthwash around in his or her mouth and send it for testing to a laboratory. What does DNA testing really tell you about your own ancestry—distant or not so distant? And most of all, how do you interpret and use the results?

Here's a letter from Dr.Mark Humphrys:
Lecturer
School of Computer Applications,
Dublin City University,
Glasnevin, Dublin 9, Ireland.

"Dear Anne:

Here's a summary of the position as I see it:

Why everybody in the west is descended from Charlemagne:

We all know that all humans are related. So a good question is: When was our Most Recent Common Ancestor (MRCA)?

Surprisingly, the answer to that question is a lot more recent than DNA studies would suggest, since we are searching all lines of descent, rather than just the lines genes traveled on. You do not inherit all of your ancestor's DNA, but only a small part of it. And yet, even if you inherit NONE of their DNA (which is not only possible, but probable, as you go back far enough), they are still your ancestor.

To find the answer to the MRCA, we need to look beyond DNA studies. Mathematical models suggest that, if humans picked mates randomly, the MRCA is in historical times, perhaps c. 1200 AD! This is an amazing result, suggesting that we do not have to go back into prehistory to find an ancestor of every single human! But obviously humans do not pick mates randomly—they tend to mate with people in their local geographic area.

Computer simulations that take this into account suggest that even with a high degree of local mating, the MRCA is still in historical times, perhaps c. 300 AD. If we consider just the West, the MRCA may be as recent as c. 1000 AD.

How realistic are these models?

Well, there has been a growing collection of REAL, proven descents from medieval figures in genealogy. For instance, my own children have proven descents—through many different lines—from Charlemagne, who lived around 800 AD. He is the ancestor of most of the royal houses of Europe and so is a natural focal point for the genealogies of the West.

My web page, Royal Descents of Famous People, is a large and growing list of famous people in the West who are all proven descendants of Charlemagne. And if all these people have proven descents, every step of the way, how many more people must have descents in reality that cannot be proved because of the scarcity of records? It must be a much greater number. My work is a strong indicator that everyone in the West descends from medieval royalty.

In short, work by a number of people—my genealogical study, other people's computer simulations and mathematical models—all confirm each other's findings that the MRCA for a large, interbreeding area such as the West, is within recent recorded history. Another finding of those models is that not long before the MRCA, if someone is the ancestor of anyone alive today, they are the ancestor of all people alive today. Since Charlemagne is probably around that early date for the West, and since he is a proven ancestor of some people, it is likely that he is the ancestor of all people in the West.

Everybody in the West is descended from Charlemagne:

In conclusion, if you have west European ancestry at all, it seems virtually impossible for you not to be descended from Charlemagne, who lived around 800 AD. 90 percent of the world (including all the West) is descended from Confucius:

For the MRCA of the whole world, we need to consider extremely isolate aboriginal populations. If they were truly isolated, we may have to go back thousands of years to get a common ancestor with them. For people who did not live in isolated enclaves though—the West, Middle East, more or less all of Asia, most of Africa—the MRCA is highly likely to be in recent historical times (late BC, possibly even AD). Anyone with ancestry from these areas is, for example, almost certainly a descendant of Confucius, who lived around 500 BC and who is a proven ancestor of some people alive today in China, hence probably ancestor of all people in the world except the extremely isolated.

This exciting consensus is fairly new, and is supported by three independent fields of (a) genealogy, (b) mathematical models, and (c) computer simulations.

The findings are robust with respect to barriers such as religion, class difference, outcall one needs is a tiny amount of crossing of such barriers in the population in order to get everyone today (of different religions etc.) with a recent common ancestor.

The only thing that can push back the MRCA before historical times is total geographic isolation of populations from each other, which we know did not happen for most of the world. People are inspired (rightly so) by DNA studies of ancient common human ancestors tens of thousands of years ago. And yet the fact is that we are almost certainly all descended from any historical figure in classical times that left descendants."

———
end quote
———

Web pages on MRCAs:
http://computing.dcu.ie/~humphrys/FamTree/Royal/ca.html
http://computing.dcu.ie/~humphrys/FamTree/Royal/ca.genetic.html
http://computing.dcu.ie/~humphrys/FamTree/Royal/ca.math.html
http://computing.dcu.ie/~humphrys/FamTree/Royal/famous.descents.html

The Web pages include a fantastic computer simulation by a gentleman named Rohde at MIT to work out the MRCA for a non-random mating model. He confirms much of Chang's work, and in general it is another strong indicator that the MRCA for the world (or 99 percent of it) is post-1000 BC—maybe even AD.

Regards
—Mark
Dr.Mark Humphrys

Lecturer
School of Computer Applications,
Dublin City University,
Glasnevin, Dublin 9, Ireland.
http://computing.dcu.ie/~humphrys/

E-Letter from Bryan Sykes:

From: Bryan Sykes
To: Anne Hart
Sent: Wednesday, December 01, 2004 4:28 PM

Subject: Re: Thank you for starting us to search for English ancestors

Dear Anne

Well I suppose that's what academics are for. I'm so thrilled that my research has led to something useful. It certainly didn't seem so at the time.

On a serious vein, what has happened in 'genetic genealogy' is extremely unusual. Blue sky scientific research has opened up a field which is now being championed by yourself and others. The research that counts is now being done by enthusiastic practitioners—mainly unpaid. It is the return of the long forgotten 19th century paragon—the amateur scientist. I feel a ponderous and pompous article coming on!

Best wishes—and a very happy Christmas.

Bryan

Learn to Interpret and Understand the Results of Your Own Genetic Tests

Learn to interpret the results of your own DNA test and expand your historical research ability to trace your ancestry. "An interesting idea was expressed by a colleague from Canada, Dr. Charles Scriver," explains geneticist, Dr. Batsheva Bonné-Temir. "At a meeting which I organized here in Israel on Genetic Diversity

Among Jews in 1990, Dr. Scriver gave a paper on 'What Are Genes Like that Doing in a Place Like This? Human History and Molecular Prosopography.'

He claimed that a biological trait has two histories, a biological component and a cultural component." Dr. Charles Scriver is founder of the DeBelle Laboratory of Biochemical Genetics in Canada. He also established screening programs in Montreal for thalassaemia and Tay Sachs Disease.

According to Bonné-Tamir, at the 1990 meeting in Israel on Genetic Diversity Among Jews, Dr. Charles Scriver stated, "When the event clusters and an important cause of it is biological, the cultural history also is likely to be important because it may explain why the persons carrying the gene are in the particular place at the time."

The term, "when the event clusters" refers to an event when genes cluster together in a DNA test because the genes are similar in origin, that is, they have a common ancestral origin in a particular area, a common ancestor.

"When I look at my own papers throughout the years," says Bonné-Tamir. "I find that I have been quite a pioneer in realizing the significance of combining the history of individuals or of populations with their biological attributes. This is now a leading undertaking in many studies which use, for example, mutations to estimate time to the most recent ancestors and alike."

What lines of inquiry are used in genetics? Dr. Charles R. Scriver wrote a chapter in Batsheva Bonné-Temir's book, titled *What Are Genes Like That Doing in a Place Like This? Human History and Molecular Prosopography*. The book title is: *Genetic Diversity Among Jews: Diseases and Markers at the DNA Level*. Bonné-Tamir, B. and Adam, A. Oxford University Press. 1992. With permission, an excerpt is reprinted below from page 319: "When a disease clusters in a particular community, two lines of inquiry follow:

1. Is the clustering caused by shared environmental exposure? Or is it explained by host susceptibility accountable to biological and/or cultural inheritance?

2. If the explanation is biological, how are the determinants inherited?

These lines of inquiry imply that a disease has two different histories, one biological, the other cultural. One involves genes (heredity), pathways of development (ontogeny), and constitutional factors; the other, demography, migration and cultural practice.

Neither history is mutually exclusive. Such thinking shifts the focus of inquiry from sick populations and incidence of disease to sick individuals and the cause of their particular disease. The person with the disease becomes the object of concern which is not the same as the disease the person has." (Page. 319).

Chapter Eight

Consumers Can Use Genetic Tests to Identify At-Risk Relatives

After hearing from Dr. Scriver by email, I then emailed Stanley M. Diamond. He contacted writer, Barbara Khait, and got permission for me to reprint in this book some of what she wrote about Diamond's project. It's the chapter, "*Genetics Study Identifies At-risk relatives*" from **Celebrating the Family** published by Ancestry.com Publishing.

Check out the Web site at: http://shops.ancestry.com/product.asp?productid=2625&shopid=128.

Here's the reprinted article. Persons interested may go to the Web site for more information. I found out about Stanley M. Diamond from Dr. Scriver, since he mentioned Stanley M. Diamond's project in the book chapter Scriver wrote for Batsheva Bonné-Temir's book on *Genetic Diversity Among Jews: Diseases and Markers at the DNA Level*. Barbara Khait's chapter follows.

*　　　　　　　*　　　　　　　*

"In 1977, Stanley Diamond of Montreal learned he carried the betathalassemia genetic trait. Though common among people of Mediterranean, Middle Eastern, Southeast Asian and African descent, the trait is rare among descendants of eastern European Jews like Stan. His doctor made a full study of the family and identified Stanley's father as the source.

"Stan was spurred to action by a letter his brother received in 1991 from a previously unknown first cousin. Stan asked the cousin, "Do you carry the beta-thalassemia trait?" Though the answer was no, Stan began his journey to find out what other members of his family might be unsuspecting carriers.

"Later that year, Stan found a relative from his paternal grandmother's family, the Widelitz family. Again he asked, "Is there any incidence of anemia in your family?"His newfound cousin answered, "Oh, you mean beta-thalassemia? It's all over the family!"

"There was no question now that the trait could now be traced to Stan's grandmother, Masha Widelitz Diamond and that Masha's older brother Aaron also had to have been a carrier. Stan's next question: who passed the trait onto Masha and Aaron? Was it their mother, Sura Nowes, or their father, Jankiel Widelec?

"At the 1992 annual summer seminar on Jewish genealogy in New York City, Stan conferred with Dr. Robert Desnick, who suggested that Stan's first step should be to determine whether the trait was related to a known mutation or a gene unique to his family. He advised Stan to seek out another Montrealer, Dr. Charles Scriver of McGill University—Montreal Children's Hospital. With the help of a grant, Dr. Scriver undertook the necessary DNA screening with the goal of determining the beta-thalassemia mutation.

"During this time, Stan began to research his family's history in earnest and identified their nineteenth century home town of Ostrow Mazowiecka in Poland. With the help of birth, marriage, and death records for the Jewish population of Ostrow Mazowiecka filmed by The Church of Jesus Christ of Latter-day Saints (LOS), Stan was able to construct his family tree.

"Late in 1993, Dr. Scriver faxed the news that the mutation had been identified and that it was, in fact, a novel mutation. Independently, Dr. Ariella Oppenheim at Jerusalem's Hebrew University-Hadassah Hospital mad e a similar discovery about a woman who had recently emigrated from the former Soviet Union.

"The likelihood that we were witnessing a DNA region 'identical by descent' in the two families was impressive. We had apparently discovered a familial relationship between Stanley and the woman in Jerusalem, previously unknown to either family," says Dr. Scriver.

"It wasn't very long ago when children born with thalassemia major seldom made it past the age of ten. Recent advances have increased life span but, to stay alive, these children must undergo blood transfusions every two to four weeks. And every night, they must receive painful transfusions of a special drug for up to twelve hours.

"The repeated blood transfusions lead to a buildup of iron in the body that can damage the heart, liver, and other organs. That's why, when the disease is misdiagnosed as mild chronic anemia, the prescription of additional iron is even more harmful. Right now, no cure exists for the disease, though medical experts say experimental bone-marrow transplants and gene-therapy procedures may one day lead to one.

"Stan's primary concern is that carriers of thalassemia trait may marry, often unaware that their mild chronic anemia may be something else. To aid in his search for carriers of his family's gene mutation of the beta-thalassemia trait, he founded and coordinates an initiative known as Jewish Records Indexing-Poland, an award-winning Internet-based index of Jewish vital records in Poland, with more than one million references. This database is helping Jewish families, particularly those at increased risk for hereditary conditions and diseases, trace their medical histories, as well as geneticists."

Says Dr. Robert Burk, professor of epidemiology at the Albert Einstein College of Medicine at Yeshiva University, and principal investigator for the Cancer Longevity, Ancestry and Lifestyle (CLAL) study in the Jewish population (currently focusing on prostate cancer), "Through the establishment of a searchable database from Poland, careful analysis of the relationship between individuals will be possible at both the familial and the molecular level.

"This will afford us the opportunity to learn not only more about the Creator's great work, but will also allow (us) researchers new opportunities to dissect the cause of many diseases in large established pedigrees."

Several other medical institutions, including Yale University's Cancer Genetics Program, the Epidemiology-Genetics Program at the Johns Hopkins School of Medicine, and Mount Sinai Hospital's School of Medicine have recognized Diamond's work as an outstanding application of knowing one's family history and as a guide to others who may be trying to trace their medical histories, particularly those at increased risk for hereditary conditions and diseases.

In February 1998, in a breakthrough effort, Stanley discovered another member of his family who carried the trait. He found the descendants of Jankiel's niece and nephew—first cousins who married—David Lustig and his wife, Fanny Bengelsdorf. This was no ordinary find—he located the graves by using a map of the Ostrow

Mazowiecka section of Chicago's Waldheim Cemetery and contacted the person listed as the one paying for perpetual care, David and Fanny's grandson, Alex.

"It turned out Alex, too, had been diagnosed as a beta-thalassemia carrier by his personal physician fifteen years earlier. The discovery that David and Fanny's descendants were carriers of the beta-thalassemia trait convinced Stan, Dr. Scriver, and Dr.Oppenheim that Hersz Widelec, born in 1785,must be the source of the family's novel mutation.

"'This groundbreaking work helps geneticists all over the world understand the trait and its effects on one family,' says Dr. Oppenheim.

"A most important contribution of Stanley Diamond's work is increasing the awareness among his relatives and others to the possibility that they carry a genetic trait which with proper measures, can be prevented in future generations. In addition, the work has demonstrated the power of modern genetics in identifying distant relatives, and helps to clarify how genetic diseases are being spread throughout the world."

For more information about thalassemia, contact: Cooley's Anemia Foundation (129–09 26th Avenue. Flushing, New York, 11354; by phone 800–522–7222; or online at www.cooleysanemia.org). For more about Stanley Diamond's research, visit his Web site (www.diamondgen.org).

Thalassemia is not only carried by people living today in Mediterranean lands. The first Polish (not Jewish) carrier of Beta-Thal was discovered in the last few years in Bialystok, Poland. Stanley Diamond met with the Director of the Hematology Institute in Warsaw

in November 2002, and the Director of the Hematology Institute in Warsaw indicated that they now have identified 52 carriers. Check out these Web sites listed below if the subject intrigues you.

"Genealogy with an extra reason"…Beta-Thalassemia Research Project.
http://www.diamondgen.org
JTA genetic disorder and Polish Jewish history
www.jta.org/page_view_story.asp?intarticleid=11608&intcategoryid=5
IAJGS Lifetime Achievement Award
http://www.jewishgen.org/ajgs/awards.html
Jewish Records Indexing—Poland
http://www.jri-poland.org

Chapter Nine

Understanding HLA Genes (White Blood Cells) Tissue Typing and Ethnicity

Can scientists test white blood cells, do some tissue typing, and come up with your ethnicity? HLA genes are white blood cells. Anthropologists look at white blood cells called by the scientific name of HLA genes to study genetic drift. If you have a research need to learn about tissue typing, you might want to read about understanding the HLA genes. Tissue typing is usually done on white blood cells, or leukocytes. The markers are referred to as human leukocyte antigens (HLA). A good starting point is to read the definitions and excerpts about tissue typing testing on the 'About' Health and Fitness Web site at: http://thyroid.about.com/library/immune/blimm25.htm?terms=Human+Leukocyte+Antigen.

The L in HLA stands for leukocyte/leucocyte (Gk leuko=white). A DNA test now involves only taking a sample of saliva and gently rubbing the inside of your mouth with a cotton or felt-tipped stick in the same way as you'd brush your teeth (without touching your teeth—just the inside of your cheek.) Years ago DNA tests used to involve looking at 'white' blood cells. Years ago, people would give a small blood sample (or possibly sampling a site of infection), and a trained phlebotomist would take the blood sample.

Some types of DNA tests for disease require a blood sample taken anonymously at a clinic, but for DNA tests for ancestry, you don't necessarily need to use a blood sample. Today, you can take a DNA test at home with a kit sent to you in the mail by just swapping the inside of your mouth (cheek) and sending the swab in a plastic bag or tube and regular padded mailing envelope.

The Brigham Young University (BYU) study used to have participants give blood (of which HLA typing is possibly involved). They use mouthwash collections currently. As Ugo A. Perego, MS, Senior Project Administrator, Molecular Genealogy Research Project, BYU emphasizes, "We stopped using blood a few years ago. All our collections are now based on a simple 45 seconds rinse using mouthwash."

DNA for ancestry doesn't test for disease. You can take another type of DNA test for diseases. The HLA system can provide information or guides to genetic disposition to disease. Given the apprehension about giving a cheek swab to be 'DNA tested' for the Y-chromosome, having HLA alleles typed, compared, and possibly posted to the net would discourage most people looking for genetic tests for ancestry only. So HLA testing is used by anthropologists and medical personnel for research in such topics as genetic drift or molecular anthropology.

If you ever need a tissue donor or have to get your tissue typed for medical reasons, that's when the HLA genes play a major role in tissue typing. Interestingly, when small communities are isolated for long periods of time, and bottlenecks pare down the population to only a few founders, genetic drift may occur. That's when the anthropologists and evolutionary biologists look at the HLA genes.

With some DNA testing companies offering racial percentages tests, Y-chromosome tests, and mtDNA tests, what is being done with mtDNA testing for maternal lineages? How can we trace female relatives or ancestors who leave no written records of their name or existence?

Will studies of HLA genes be used by others in various fields as research now is used by anthropologists studying genetic drift, scientists studying tissue differentiation, or physicians looking at how white cells fight infection?

Dr. Peter Reed has a PhD in Human Genetics from the University of Oxford and was a pioneer in the use of STR genetic markers in medical research. He explains here that HLA genes primarily determine how our blood cells recognize and react to other cells present in our bodies. In particular, this makes HLA genes important in how our body responds to 'foreign bodies.'

For example, the HLA genes as white blood cells fight infection. When bacteria or viruses enter our bodies, the HLA genes are there to do battle. When organs or tissue are transplanted, HLA genes have to be considered.

They would attack the foreign tissue placed in the body. "When people talk about blood typing or tissue matching, on the whole, they are referring to determining some aspect of the set of HLA genes," says Reed. "HLA genes are perhaps the most variable of all human genes. Across the population, some HLA genes have dozens of different forms of genes or 'alleles.'"

The result is that two randomly chosen people are unlikely to share identical HLA genes. "Even within families, there is a good chance that each family member has a different set of HLA genes," says Reed.

"That's why finding a 'suitable match' for a transplant can be difficult."

It's also the reason why we all react differently to infections. On the plus side, HLA genes (white blood cells) can deal with all the different infections we get during our lives, usually without being aware of them.

Apart from the obvious medical importance of a role in responding to infection and transplantation, there is another role. It's perhaps one of the primary reasons that HLA genes are some of the most intensely studied of all human genes.

"This relates to the role HLA genes play in determining how our blood cells respond to the other cells of the body," says Reed. "In certain circumstances, some of a person's own cells are mistaken as 'foreign bodies.' These cells are responded to as if they were an infection." The technical jargon for this is called auto-immunity.

"This can result in disease. This sort of problem is believed to be one of the underlying causes many fairly common diseases, more appropriately termed 'conditions'. Such conditions include Rheumatoid Arthritis and Juvenile Diabetes," says Reed. "A connection between particular types of HLA genes and certain conditions was first recognized more than thirty years ago." Since then many connections between HLA and human conditions have been identified.

These genes are obviously very important in human health, and are often suspected as being the major genetic causes of numerous conditions. Consequently, there are a number of clinical programs where HLA genes are screened (particularly in children) to research and even determine the risk of later disease.

"One aspect of the high variability of HLA genes, is that certain types (alleles) of certain HLA genes have been found to be geographically/ethnically distributed," says Reed. "For example, some alleles of some HLA genes may be more frequent in Japan than in England. Therefore there is some possible utility in the use of HLA genes in determining ancestry from different geographical locations. However, because the HLA genes are only a small fraction of all our genes, examining HLA genes alone is not likely to be very informative."

"Because HLA genes, like almost all our other genes, are shuffled and mixed as they are passed on from parents to children, it's difficult to determine the exact set of HLA genes of even one or two generations previous," Reed says. "So they have little utility in determining recent ancestry."

There could be some utility of HLA for genealogy. "This could be so in certain circumstances," Reed explains, "but the hurdles mentioned above will need to be overcome. I'm exploring this further."

According to Ann Turner, Genealogy-DNA List Administrator, at: http://lists.rootsweb.com/index/other/Miscellaneous/GENEALOGYDNA.html, an excellent Web site for explaining HLA is located at the Web site: http://www.med.umich.edu/trans/public/hla/hla_&_you.html.

"This HLA Web site diagrams the inheritance patterns. It says HLA is on gene 6, but it means chromosome 6," reports Turner. "You also can learn about linkage disequilibrium at this site. Some genes in the HLA system are close to one another. That makes the alleles, which are a form of a gene, also linked together closely and inherited as one unit, or haplotype."

That's the original context for the word 'haplotype.' Also look at: http://www.hokkaido.bc.jrc.or.jp/laboratory/laboratory500_eng.htm, Turner notes.

*   *   *

How many DNA testing companies will show you how to interpret DNA test results for family history or direct you to instructional materials after you have had your DNA tested? Choose a company based on previous customer satisfaction, number of markers tested, and whether the company gives you choices of how many markers you want, various ethnic and geographic databases, and surname projects based on DNA-driven genealogy.

Before you select a company to test your DNA, find out how many genetic markers will be tested. For the maternal line, 400 base pairs of sequences are the minimum. For the paternal line (men only) 37 markers are great, but 25 markers also should be useful.

Some companies offer a 12-marker test for surname genealogy groups at a special price. When you order a home testing kit, you'll get mouthwash or a felt tip to rub inside your cheek and mail back. Find out how long the turnaround time is for waiting to receive your results. What is the reputation of the company? Do they have a contract with a university lab or a private lab? Who does the testing and who is the chief geneticist at their laboratory?

What research articles, if any, has that scientist written or what research studies on DNA have been performed by the person in charge of the DNA testing at the laboratory? Who owns the DNA business that contracts with the lab? How involved in genealogy-related DNA projects and databases or services is the owner?

Find a Mentor or Educational Web Site/Discussion Group on DNA Research

It's good to have a mentor to answer questions about your test results until you are able to do your own research on the Web. If you're a lay person, where can you learn enough molecular genetics to get a handle on DNA test results and untangle ancestral roots? If you've ever wondered why your genes are not where you thought they were supposed to be (in geographic location on a map), that topic of research is called molecular prosopography. See the Web site: www.linacre.ox.ac.uk/research/prosop/prosopo.stm.

Research the Social History of DNA-Driven Genealogy and Online Preventive Medicine Genetic Testing Marketed to General Consumers

Prosopography is an independent science of social history embracing genealogy, onomastics and demography. Prosopography is all about human history and genes that travel because your genes have both a cultural and a biological component. The cultural component includes onomastics which is the study of the origin of a name and its geographical and historical utilization.

Onomastics includes the study of how and when place-names were originated and used. Then there's toponymics. Toponymics is the study of names related to a place or region. See http://libraryweb.utep.edu/onomastics.html or http://www.kami.demon.co.uk/gesithas/biblio/bib08.html. And you probably know demography, is the interdisciplinary study of human populations. Demography deals with social characteristics of the population and their development.

So you'd find more information on demography by researching population studies. Phenomics is the science of customizing, tailoring, and individualizing medicines and other health treatments to the total human genome of one person.

The age of one medicine or hormone fits all is gone. As a tool, phenomics also can be applied to herbal remedies, food supplements, vitamins and minerals, hormones, and other formulas adjusted to an individual's total genome.

If you have a genetic risk for a certain disease, perhaps you can find out what way there is to prevent it by using phenomics as a tool for customizing your treatment or working on prevention strategies of lifestyle, diet, or medicine. Within phemomics, the study of customizing healthcare and treatment to your genetic signature or genetic expression is the specialized field of pharmacogenetics—the study of how to avoid adverse drug reactions based on looking at how your genes respond to various medicines or dosages of drugs.

Family history DNA testing is a new way to approach biological research. Genealogy and genetics are forms of hunting and gathering that persist. First you start with transcribed oral history. We are foragers in molecular family history.

Molecular genealogy uses DNA testing (human genetics) as a tool for untangling ancestral and recent family roots. Here's an introduction to family DNA testing to be used with oral history gathering and genealogy. Start your family history time capsule, gift basket, scrapbook, genetic genealogy, or begin a small business publicizing DNA testing for genealogy. The place for genetic genealogy is in an archives, library, museum, or good storage place.

Future generations need a DNA history of as many ancestors as they can find willing to participate and to create oral histories. Genetics is the most mathematical/statistical of the biological sciences. We have fields such as bioinformatics that combine computers and biological information. Family historians need a bridge to fill the gap between such a mathematical science as genetics and genealogy, often based on records and oral histories.

The oral history would be transcribed on acid-free paper in hard, bound copy. Photos and other memorabilia could be added. Then the basic archive would be copied onto disks such as a CD, DVD, or other, stored in a computer and on video and audio tape.

Another copy would be saved as a multimedia presentation with text, sound, voice, photos, illustrations, and video/audio and saved on a disk to be played on screen with a home entertainment player or in a computer.

You could put a smaller file online on a Web site. This molecular biography would represent not only the life of a person, but a history of the person's DNA test results, racial percentages, ethnicity, if known, and anything else about the DNA sequence as far as geographic location or even medical history, if desired, in a more private file for relatives. This is where genetics joins with genealogy.

We not only have a family history to archive, but now a genome, or at least a record of the matrilineal and patrilineal ancestry by DNA. We have the markers and the sequences. The idea is to learn enough about DNA testing and genealogy to understand what those sequences and markers mean.

What can we learn about ancestry through the mitochondrial DNA (for women and men) the Y chromosome only for men, and other markers on the genome? What should we look at to view the percentages of races such as Native American, African, East Asian, or Indo—European (Europe, Middle East, and India)?

What do these sequences tell us about our ancestry? If there's no such thing as race, what geographic locations of our ancestors are we viewing back in time when we look at the genetic markers?

What dates are we looking at—a few generations ago or 21,000 years? What do our transitions and mutations mean over a long span of time? What foods, medicines, therapies, and climates are best for our customized, individual molecular profiles?

How do we read and interpret those genetic markers? Where does genealogy and oral history fit in? Family history—genealogy—now has joined up with molecular genetics and evolutionary anthropology. And included with genealogy is the tradition of transcribing and recording oral history, diary journaling and restoration, time capsules, biography, scrap booking, videography, and photography.

The genome has reached the genealogist. Family history today is multimedia and molecular, historical and futuristic. "Progress in our knowledge of the genome and of its function has been extremely rapid since the development, in the mid-eighties, of the Polymerase Chain Reaction," says Professor of Genetics,

Guido Barbujani, (Department of Biology, University of Ferrara, Italy.) Dipartimento di Biologia, Universita' di Ferrara via L. Borsari 46, I—44100 Ferrara, Italia. See his Web site at:
http://www.unife.it/genetica/Guido/Guido.html.

Dr. Barbujani's fields of interest include human population and molecular genetics and evolution, and I've read many of his articles in the various journals of genetics and research books, such as Archaeogenetics: DNA and the population prehistory of Europe published by the McDonald Institute Monographs.

"By that method, minimal quantities of DNA can be studied, which has opened the field for a number of previously hard-to-imagine applications, ranging from gene therapy to the prediction of interactions among genes, from the sequencing of entire genomes to the retrieval of DNA sequences from extinct organisms," Barbujani explains.

"DNA technologies proved so powerful that people tend to forget about their limitations. Still, limitations exist, especially in the field of genealogical reconstructions, and future technical advancements are unlikely to be of great help.

"Consider this: Each of us has two parents, four grandparents, eight grand-grandparents, and so on. In principle, only ten generations ago (around 1750 AD) we had 1024 different ancestors. In fact, chances are our ancestors were less than 1024, because consanguineous marriages likely occurred at various stages. But even if we had only 200 independent ancestors ten generations ago, each of them contributed to our 30,000 or so genes.

"On the other hand, only one of them transmitted to us her mitochondrial DNA and, if we are males, from only one of them did we inherit our Y chromosome," Barbujani reveals. "The other 198 or 199 ancestors' contributions to our genotype are of course equally important, but there is no easy way to figure them out."

"Indeed, at every generation recombination created new associations of genes along our chromosomes, except for the mitochondrial DNA and for part of the Y chromosome, which do not recombine. In this way, traits of DNA coming from different ancestors have been assembled in a mosaic that cannot be disentangled a posteriori, in which each piece has a different, and possibly very different, origin. In short, it is an illusion to think that our mitochondrial DNA (or our Y chromosome) may allow us to understand our family history.

"These are small parts of our genome, and hence contain information on but a small bit of our biological history," says Barbujani. "Other ancestors have transmitted to us many more genes than the ancestors from whom we inherited our mitochondrial DNA, and they may have come from different parts of the world."

"That may sound frustrating to some, but population genetics has something important to tell us in this regard. Population histories are much easier to reconstruct than individual histories, because chance phenomena have a much greater impact on the latter.

"When a large number of individuals are jointly analyzed, rather robust evolutionary inferences may be drawn, even if some members of the sample have had an unusual family history. By combining measures of genetic diversity, among populations and among individuals, with the evidence coming from mitochondrial and Y-chromosome genealogies, population geneticists have shown very clearly that each population contains a large proportion of all humankind's alleles, around 85 percent, on average.

"This finding has several implications. One is: should most humans disappear because of some global catastrophe, and should only one community survive, the loss of genetic diversity would be very limited, around 15 percent. That might or might not be reassuring, but is true.

"Secondly, although many tend to think that humans come in clear racial clusters, that is not true; if, on average, populations contain 85 percent of the global human diversity, two individuals from very distant localities can be just 15 percent more different genetically than members of the same population (unless the latter are relatives, of course).

Third, if genetic diversity is so high among members of the same population, the only possible explanation is that those populations incorporated, through time, contributions from other populations at a rather high rate.

"In other words, our ancestors spent most of their evolutionary time in communities connected by extensive migratory exchanges, and not in isolated groups. Through migration, alleles of African, Asian and European origin ended up all over the world, and no biologically recognizable race evolved in our species. Therefore, it is impossible to define our origin by studying our DNA, but if it were possible, we would probably find that our roots are spread over much of the world.

"As Jonathan Marks remarked, today convincing people that there is no such thing as a human race is probably as difficult as, in the 17th century, to convince people that the earth rotates around the sun and not vice versa. However, this is a scientific fact, and perhaps the single most significant result of human evolutionary studies. Everybody can tell a Nigerian from a Japanese person, but if we move from Nigeria to Japan we shall never find a sharp boundary separating two well-distinct groups.

"Rather, we shall notice that the genetic features of people change continuously, in a gradient, and that each community harbors substantial biological differences among its members. The best way to summarize these concepts, I think, is by a slogan invented by the French anthropologist André Langaney: Tous parents, tous différents. We are all relatives, and we are all different."

Gene Power through Smarter Foods and Family History

Where can you get more information on health statistics? How can you find out more about how health statistics and statistics from research studies can be manipulated? How do you know what studies hold up and which studies are flawed or about the credibility of those who say a study is flawed? You can search sites such as the following: The National Center for Health Statistics in Hyattsville, Maryland is also on the World Wide Web at: http://www.cdc.gov/nchs/howto/w2w/newyork.htm.

What if you are doing genealogy research along with nutritional research or family medical history research and need a marriage certificate to find a relative's maiden name? For example, to view an address where to write to in order to purchase a copy of a marriage certificate for New York State, the Web site will help provide information as to where to write to in order to purchase copies of marriage licenses for New York, for example, from the year 1880 forward.

For other states, check the Web site at The National Center for Health Statistics under each state. You can also search foreign countries for records. You could also look at the Ellis Islands records, if a relative came to Ellis Island, and even view a picture of the ship at the Ellis Island Online Web site at: http://www.ellisisland.org/.

One good place to start is http://www.cdc.gov/nchs/products.htm. For publications and products, click on http://www.cdc.gov/nchs/nvss.htm for Vital Statistics. Click here http://www.cdc.gov/nchs/releases/96facts/mardiv.htm for marriage and divorce statistics.

DNA Testing Companies That Report on Deep, Ancient Maternal and Paternal Lineages: MtDNA and Y-Chromosome Testing

Companies That Bring the Power of DNA Technology to Your Home:
The DNA Testing Companies of Interest to Family Historians and Genealogists

"The Power of DNA Technology in Every Home" is the slogan of the GeneTree DNA Testing Center that supplies DNA testing applications directly to the consumer. "We would like to demonstrate how we provide the science of DNA analysis applications directly to the consumer, allowing them to conduct their own research projects in the comfort of their own home," says Terrence C. Carmichael, MS, founder of GeneTree DNA Testing Center.

"By examining the Autosomal STRs, Y-chromosome STRs and mtDNA sequence analysis and RFLP, GeneTree is helping people (such as genealogists, anthropologists, and just those generally interested) uncover their deep ancestral

migration patterns, establish biological relationships with relatives 1–50 generations apart, and uncover the mysteries of past and present relationships.

"These services are wonderful, and prove to be of great value to the consumer,
whether it is for immigration purposes, assistance with genealogy or anthropology
research, or for answering the simplest of questions, such as 'are you my father?'"

After receiving his MS degree, Carmichael went on to receive a Professional
Designation in Marketing and Sales from UCLA. Terry has worked at the DNA
laboratory bench for 4 years and spent 9 years providing Product Development,
Technical Consulting, and Marketing for the DNA purification industry, working for companies such as Bio-Rad and QIAGEN. In 2000, Carmichael co-
authored a book titled, "*How to DNA Test your Family Relationships.*"

Having started 2 successful businesses, Terry is a visionary. He has applications
submitted for 2 separate patents; one for applying DNA profiles to identification
cards and the other for a new high-throughput DNA purification product held
by Bio-Rad Laboratories.

Consumer's Guide to the Human Genome

"The human genome is about 3 x 109 base pairs long, which would weigh
about 40 pg picograms: 1 pg=10–12 grams) per genome," reports Michael
Onken. And this description appears on the science Web site of Ricky J. Sethi,
MadSci.ORG Administrator at MadSci.ORG, at the Washington University
School of Medicine. See the Web site at: at: http://www.madsci.org.

"Human cells are diploid, i.e. each contains two copies of the genome, so the
nuclear DNA from a human cell would weigh about 80 pg. If we want total cellular DNA, then we need to include mitochondrial DNA (mtDNA).

"The human mitochondrial genome is about 16,000 base pairs long. There are
about 10 copies of the genome per mitochondrion, and there are on the order of
1,000 mitochondria per cell. This gives us about 0.2 pg of mtDNA per human cell.

"There are on the order of 1014 cells per adult human, many of which are
without nuclei, like skin cells and red blood cells. This would give us just under a
kilogram of chromosomal DNA and on the order of a few grams of mitochondrial DNA in the average human body."

(This excerpt above is reprinted with permission of Ricky J. Sethi,
MadSci.ORG Administrator, at the Washington University School of Medicine.
See the Web site at http://www.madsci.org/ .)

Knowing how many genes a human has in the future will help not only
genealogists and other family and oral historians trace ancestors and keep records
of lineages, but physicians will be able to tailor medicines to help people based on

how their individual genes react to different elixirs, drugs, natural supplements, herbs, foods, and medicines.

Combined with the knowledge of rainforest tropical plants and their cures, the human genome is headed towards individualization and customization, with an appropriate mixture of food, medicine, or therapy based on one's individual genetic makeup.

To the person without a science background, knowing one's genes also is a way to connect people to their common ancestors and to those descendants. Family history can be researched not only for medical reasons, but for historical reasons, and to show how people are related to one another down through the ages. Below are the Web sites for some of the products offered by GeneTree DNA Testing Center.

GeneTree Products:
http://www.genetree.com/servlet/moonshine/goto?page_url=/products/product-groups.jsp
Y-Chromosome Information:
http://www.genetree.com/servlet/moonshine/goto?page_url=/products/product.jsp&id=7
mtDNA Information:
http://www.genetree.com/servlet/moonshine/goto?page_url=/products/product.jsp&id=8
Native American Assessment:
http://www.genetree.com/servlet/moonshine/goto?page_url=/products/product.jsp&id=20
Biography: Terrence C. Carmichael, MS
Terrence Carmichael, MS
(888) 404-GENE (ext. 207)

GeneTree DNA Testing Center
3150 Almaden Expressway, #203
San Jose, CA 95118–1253
Phone: (888) 404-GENE, (408) 723–2670
Fax: (408) 723–2671 http://www.genetree.com/
****

Chapter Ten

Finnish Genes

Check out the Discover magazine article, *Finland's Fascinating Genes, Learning Series: Genes, Race, and Medicine [Part 2]*, According to the article, "The people in this land of lakes and forests are so alike that scientists can filter out the genes that contribute to heart disease, diabetes, and asthma," by Jeff Wheelwright, DISCOVER Vol. 26 No. 04 | April 2005 | Biology & Medicine.

The UCLA study also might help you learn more about your Finn-American medical heritage. For example, Karelians from Eastern Finland and Karelia are being compared in studies to people from Western Finland to see whether or not there are any genetic predispositions in the Eastern Finns and Karelians compared to the Western Finns.

The article notes that Karelians and Eastern Finns with short arms and legs may have genes for different genetic predispositions compared to Western Finns with longer arms and legs, but all this is currently under study. Gene hunters described in the spring 1999 UCLA magazine article at: http://www.magazine.ucla.edu/year1999/spring99_03.html and http://www.magazine.ucla.edu/year1999/spring99_03_02.html state that Leena Peltonen, of the world's foremost geneticists, helped to put Finland on the map as a global powerhouse in genetic research. She hopes to do the same for UCLA.

Finland has a small population, isolation, and less immigration than other European nations. The government kept meticulous tax records. As a result, Finland has medical records on individuals that go back more than three hundred years.

With carefully written medical and genealogical records, it's one way to trace familial health and ailments as well as family surnames. According to the UCLA 1999 magazine article, "Finland also has a system of free, high-quality health care in which patients trust their doctors and are highly willing to participate in medical research."

According to the UCLA magazine article, "In the 20 years that she has been studying genetic defects, Peltonen has identified no fewer than 18 genes related to such common disorders as multiple sclerosis and schizophrenia as well as more obscure diseases like AGT, a rare and horrific brain disorder found almost only among children in Finland."

In 1998, Peltonen localized the gene for familial combined hyperlipidemia, or FCHL, in a group of Finnish families. According to the UCLA magazine article, "the condition leads to the early onset of coronary-artery disease, which remains one of the leading causes of death in the industrialized world."

Check out the UCLA Human Genetics Web site at: http://www.genetics.ucla.edu/home/future.htm. Or if you're in the Los Angeles area, you can hear guest speakers presented by the Department of Human Genetics, David Geffen School of Medicine at UCLA. In your own area, go the many free lectures on genetics open to the public and learn what scientists are talking about in the fields of human genetic variation, population structure, or temperature sensation.

How can you (as a general consumer) apply what scientists have learned yesterday to benefit humanity today? For example, Peltonen's findings on FCHL coincided with a study by UCLA geneticist Jake Lusis, who localized the same gene using a mouse model. "The two scientists, who only learned of each other's research when each published a paper in the same issue of Nature Genetics, are now working together," according to the UCLA magazine article of 1999 titled *Gene Hunter*. You'll find the entire article on the Web site at: http://www.magazine.ucla.edu/year1999/spring99_03.html.

Check out this 1999 article as well as the more recent April 2005 issue of *Discover* magazine article which also describes Peltonen's more recent work at UCLA in genetic research and particularly with Finnish genes. You'll find that the Internet's Web can act as a springboard to motivate you as a consumer with no science background to read about what is being done in the evolving field of genetic testing.

If several scientists can collaborate, so can a world of consumers. Your goal would be to find out how to interpret and apply the results of any genetic tests to improve your quality of life and health. You don't need a science degree to move into new areas. Scientists are doing this daily.

Consumers need to observe the proliferation of information available online and in libraries. Federal research and the Human Genome Project have been mapping human genes since 1990. Ever since the human genome code was cracked in 2000, a flood of publications, articles, books, DNA testing companies, DNA testing kits, and DNA-driven genealogy services proliferated. What's offered as a result of testing is information. For every gene hunter, there is or could be a consumer seeking practical applications of such research.

Genetics is about preventive medicine. As a consumer, you've got breadth. Scientists have depth. They are only beginning to collaborate with one another and get the breadth that general consumers always had without much science knowledge. Genetics is a horizontal expression of a vertical desire. The consumer represents the horizontal breadth of knowledge.

The scientist's hierarchy sits amidst the vertical tower of scientific terminology. It's about language and communication as much as it's about science. Consumers want tests interpreted in plain language so they can readily apply the results to change their lifestyle.

Do scientists working in different disciplines really collaborate with one another? They have to now that the consumer is involved in the practical side of genetics—information dissemination. Collaboration means understanding how to interpret your test results and apply the research to what nourishes your body.

Chapter Eleven

What's the Consumer's Watchdog Role?

What should the consumer emphasize when seeking involvement in the nutritional genomics arena or in looking at DNA testing for ancestry for practical applications beyond genealogy or archaeogenetics? Look where the money is being spent. More money is spent on advertising for cereals in the United States than is spent by the government on education, according to a video aired July 23, 2003 at television's History Channel titled "American Eats."

Do you eat or remember the typical American diet that includes the old favorites such as Jell-o, Spam, Hershey bars, frozen TV dinners by Swanson and Birdseye, won-ton soup, kielbasa, pizza, pasta, feta cheese, dolmas, and cotton candy? I grew up on those products in the early fifties—in the heart of Brooklyn's Little Italy and Greektown, where the "Mediterranean diet" (Med Diet)—hummos on pita bread competed with spaghetti and tomato sauce and chow mein to go competed with Spam and Twinkies. The old-fashioned typical American diet, influenced by a variety of diverse immigrants gave all of us choices in what foods we ate. Still, we all had food habits and customs that tweaked our core identity or ethnic ancestry in a snack-based world.

Some people still can't view a movie at home or in a theatre without buying snacks and liquid candy-type soda, caffeinated or similar beverages. Some body types use caffeine instead of mild exercise to become more alert. Others use a sugar jolt from a bolt of insulin and adrenalin. And some genotypes are so overaroused by sensitized nervous systems that one spoonful of sugar or honey or a sip of caffeine causes a panic attack.

A combination of watching horror films and snacking on candy in the movies during the fifties was too much for many delicate nervous systems. Today children are overwhelmed by movie or video special effects that toss their brain and heart rhythms out of sync, sometimes into seizures. Children still drink sugary fruit juices, and the diabetes epidemic is growing, especially among minorities.

When I grew up in the fifties, convenience was king, and we ate the food introduced by all the immigrant groups. In September 1953, I'd come home from seventh grade to a frozen Swanson's turkey TV dinner or a burger with mayo, tomato and lettuce on a bun and mashed potatoes followed by a pint of mint chip ice cream almost every day. How about you? There's no way I'm eating like that today. View the excellent videos on American Eats and More American Eats available from http://www.historychannel.com/.

Think about high advertising budgets for snacks advertised a decade ago. What is frequently advertised on TV currently? Drugs—medicines for colds, flu, allergies, high cholesterol, arthritis, and most other chronic illnesses related to years of eating the wrong foods for your genotype. Think of advertising geared to aging boomers. Then there's the shock advertising that jolts you from your alpha state of meditation with loud ambulance sirens and shouts of illness, advertising designed to whip fear into an aging population in order to sell anything from devices to call for emergency help to medicines, through either shock, fear, concern, or worry.

It seems as if most TV commercials today either show people with illness or allergy, or the ads are about drugs for chronic illnesses from high cholesterol to arthritis. Could those chronic illnesses have occurred partly as the result of a one diet-fits-all marketing mentality? You don't see any TV ads yet on eating according to your genotype.

Let's see what pops up in the future. Healthcare in advertising is big business. You do see more ads for drugs and exercise equipment, air filters, and emergency electronic response equipment than you do for snacks nowadays, except on the children's shows and cartoons.

Infomercials on exercise equipment run all night along with ads for emergency electronic response communications devices that use shock advertising to scare the wits out of older adults—ambulance sirens, people shouting for help, an opening scene of a white-haired person collapsed on the floor. It certainly frightens older people into changing the station to something less disturbing. These ads come on in the middle of the news, as if the news wasn't stressful enough to watch, but also appear all night long just when older adults who can't sleep are looking for comforting scenes to watch for relaxation.

Think about the old cigarette ads of the fifties on television now replaced by ads for asthma drugs, diabetes blood testing equipment, pet medicines, even vitamins, but vitamins geared for older adults. All those illnesses we see dozens of times a day in the television ads, could they be due to eating the wrong foods or remaining too sedentary? For some genotypes exercise can do more harm than moderate walking a half hour to an hour a day. The food and the exercise would need to be tailored to your body. What about lifestyle changes or stress levels?

Does your body secrete too much stress hormones such as cortisol when you exercise? Changes in diet may not be enough if you're being abused daily by someone, either psychologically, financially, physically, emotionally, or sexually. Maybe you're not allowed to turn on the air conditioner at home or the heat because you're married to someone in good health who's so thrifty that your health isn't being taken into account. Be aware of the variables.

Consider the effects that widespread sugar use had on teeth and on diabetes II among minorities, children, obese persons, and older adults. Is it your food, a virus, or your genes, that contribute to obesity? Are you addicted to the sugar in your cereals, in your "alternative to dairy" beverages? Have you measured the surge of sugar in your bloodstream after drinking a glass of soy, almond, oat, or rice milk with added sweeteners? Is anyone out there drinking Noni juice? I am, by the case, two tablespoons full daily.

Do you make your own unprocessed alternative to dairy products? How do they affect your health? Is your diet too high in soy? Could it be affecting your thyroid? Or is the mercury in the fish you eat causing nervous system problems and hair loss? Have you tried a type of fish less known to have contamination of mercury in amounts unsafe to humans? Do you reach for a can of soda instead of filtered water? Are pesticides affecting your nervous system? How important is convenience for you?

More employers are trimming retiree health care insurance coverage. The cost of providing prescription medicine for older adults is urgent. In light of this, many are turning toward nutritional and genetic research solutions in hope of preventing the need for many different, costly, and sometimes interacting pre-scription medicines in old age.

Consumers can research studies and information from their Congressional Budget Office. Also see studies such as the one released on July 23, 2003, from the University of Maryland, School of Pharmacy that found in the year 2000 only 39 percent of people ages 65 to 69 in the USA had health care insurance from their employers. Coverage is dropping. Is there a nutritional genomic alter-native? If your insurance coverage stops upon retirement, can better choices of food play a role in keeping you healthier longer? It's all about choices.

Directory of DNA-Testing Companies

Family Tree DNA

1. Family Tree DNA—Genealogy by Genetics, Ltd.
World Headquarters
1919 North Loop West, Suite 110 Houston, Texas 77008, USA.
http://www.familytreedna.com/

2. Trace Genetics LLC
PO Box 2010
Davis, CA 95617
http://www.tracegenetics.com

3. DNA Direct, Inc.
Pier 9—Suite 105
San   Francisco,   CA   94111   USA,   Customer   Service,   Toll   Free:
1–877–646–0222, Main Office, Phone: 415–646–0222
Fax: 415–646–0224, Web: http://www.dnadirect.com/

4. Title: Paternity DNA Testing By paternitytesters.com. *Description:*
Paternitytesters.com—Paternity Testing Laboratory offering AABB DNA
Paternity Testing, Cheap Prices & Free DNA Banking Worldwide. For
Confidential Results in 5 days, call 866–273–8323.

5. AncestryByDNA
http://www.ancestrybydna.com/

6. DNAPrint Genomics
http://www.dnaprint.com/
DNAPrint Genomics, Inc.
900 Cocoanut Avenue
Sarasota, Florida 34236

Appendix A

Dictionary of Genetic Terms

Reprinted with the permission of the Human Genome Project.

The **online** updated presentation of this publication is a special feature of the Human Genome Project Information Web site **Dictionary of Genetic Terms at: http://www.doegenomes.org/.**

The Human Genome Project Web site also has links to numerous audio, video, and educational materials. Also see the genetics glossary at: http://doegenomestolife. org/glossary/glossary.shtml.

Dictionary of Genetic Terms

Genomics and Its Impact on Medicine and Society: A 2001 Primer

A

Acquired genetic mutation
> *See:* somatic cell genetic mutation

Additive genetic effects
> When the combined effects of alleles at different loci are equal to the sum of their individual effects.
> *See also:* anticipation, complex trait

Adenine (A)
> A nitrogenous base, one member of the base pair AT (adenine-thymine).
> *See also:* base pair, nucleotide

Affected relative pair

Individuals related by blood, each of whom is affected with the same trait. Examples are affected sibling, cousin, and avuncular pairs.

See also: avuncular relationship

Aggregation technique

A technique used in model organism studies in which embryos at the 8-cell stage of development are pushed together to yield a single embryo (used as an alternative to microinjection).

See also: model organisms

Allele

Alternative form of a genetic locus; a single allele for each locus is inherited from each parent (e.g., at a locus for eye color the allele might result in blue or brown eyes).

See also: locus, gene expression

Allogeneic

Variation in alleles among members of the same species.

Alternative splicing

Different ways of combining a gene's exons to make variants of the complete protein

Amino acid

Any of a class of 20 molecules that are combined to form proteins in living things. The sequence of amino acids in a protein and hence protein function are determined by the genetic code.

Amplification

An increase in the number of copies of a specific DNA fragment; can be in vivo or in vitro.

See also: cloning, polymerase chain reaction

Animal model

See: model organisms

Annotation

Adding pertinent information such as gene coded for, amino acid sequence, or other commentary to the database entry of raw sequence of DNA bases.

See also: bioinformatics

Anticipation

Each generation of offspring has increased severity of a genetic disorder; e.g., a grandchild may have earlier onset and more severe symptoms than the parent, who had earlier onset than the grandparent.

See also: additive genetic effects, complex trait

Antisense

Nucleic acid that has a sequence exactly opposite to an mRNA molecule made by the body; binds to the mRNA molecule to prevent a protein from being made.

See also: transcription

Apoptosis

Programmed cell death, the body's normal method of disposing of damaged, unwanted, or unneeded cells.

See also: cell

Arrayed library

Individual primary recombinant clones (hosted in phage, cosmid, YAC, or other vector) that are placed in two-dimensional arrays in microtiter dishes. Each primary clone can be identified by the identity of the plate and the clone location (row and column) on that plate. Arrayed libraries of clones can be used for many applications, including screening for a specific gene or genomic region of interest.

See also: library, genomic library, gene chip technology

Assembly

Putting sequenced fragments of DNA into their correct chromosomal positions.

Autoradiography

A technique that uses X-ray film to visualize radioactively labeled molecules or fragments of molecules; used in analyzing length and number of DNA fragments after they are separated by gel electrophoresis.

Autosomal dominant

A gene on one of the non-sex chromosomes that is always expressed, even if only one copy is present. The chance of passing the gene to offspring is 50% for each pregnancy.

See also: autosome, dominant, gene

Autosome

A chromosome not involved in sex determination. The diploid human genome consists of a total of 46 chromosomes: 22 pairs of autosomes, and 1 pair of sex chromosomes (the X and Y chromosomes).

See also: sex chromosome

Avuncular relationship

The genetic relationship between nieces and nephews and their aunts and uncles.

B

Backcross

A cross between an animal that is heterozygous for alleles obtained from two parental strains and a second animal from one of those parental strains. Also used to describe the breeding protocol of an outcross followed by a backcross.

See also: model organisms

Bacterial artificial chromosome (BAC)

A vector used to clone DNA fragments (100-to 300-kb insert size; average, 150 kb) in *Escherichia coli* cells. Based on naturally occurring F-factor plasmid found in the bacterium *E. coli*.

See also: cloning vector

Bacteriophage

See: phage

Base

One of the molecules that form DNA and RNA molecules.

See also: nucleotide, base pair, base sequence

Base pair (bp)

Two nitrogenous bases (adenine and thymine or guanine and cytosine) held together by weak bonds. Two strands of DNA are held together in the shape of a double helix by the bonds between base pairs.

Base sequence

The order of nucleotide bases in a DNA molecule; determines structure of proteins encoded by that DNA.

Base sequence analysis

A method, sometimes automated, for determining the base sequence.

Behavioral genetics

The study of genes that may influence behavior.

Bioinformatics

The science of managing and analyzing biological data using advanced computing techniques. Especially important in analyzing genomic research data.

See also: informatics

Bioremediation

The use of biological organisms such as plants or microbes to aid in removing hazardous substances from an area.

Biotechnology

A set of biological techniques developed through basic research and now applied to research and product development. In particular, biotechnology refers to the use by industry of recombinant DNA, cell fusion, and new bioprocessing techniques.

Birth defect

Any harmful trait, physical or biochemical, present at birth, whether a result of a genetic mutation or some other nongenetic factor.

See also: congenital, gene, mutation, syndrome

BLAST

A computer program that identifies homologous (similar) genes in different organisms, such as human, fruit fly, or nematode.

C

Cancer

Diseases in which abnormal cells divide and grow unchecked. Cancer can spread from its original site to other parts of the body and can be fatal.

See also: hereditary cancer, sporadic cancer

Candidate gene

A gene located in a chromosome region suspected of being involved in a disease.

See also: positional cloning, protein

Capillary array

Gel-filled silica capillaries used to separate fragments for DNA sequencing. The small diameter of the capillaries permit the application of higher electric fields, providing high speed, high throughput separations that are significantly faster than traditional slab gels.

Carcinogen

Something which causes cancer to occur by causing changes in a cell's DNA.

See also: mutagene

Carrier

An individual who possesses an unexpressed, recessive trait.

cDNA library

A collection of DNA sequences that code for genes. The sequences are generated in the laboratory from mRNA sequences.

See also: messenger RNA

Cell

The basic unit of any living organism that carries on the biochemical processes of life.

See also: genome, nucleus

Centimorgan (cM)

A unit of measure of recombination frequency. One centimorgan is equal to a 1% chance that a marker at one genetic locus will be separated from a marker at a second locus due to crossing over in a single generation. In human beings, one centimorgan is equivalent, on average, to one million base pairs.

See also: megabase

Centromere

A specialized chromosome region to which spindle fibers attach during cell division.

Chimera (pl. chimaera)

An organism that contains cells or tissues with a different genotype. These can be mutated cells of the host organism or cells from a different organism or species.

Chimeraplasty

An experimental targeted repair process in which a desirable sequence of DNA is combined with RNA to form a chimeraplast. These molecules bind selectively to the target DNA. Once bound, the chimeraplast activates a naturally occurring gene-correcting mechanism. Does not use viral or other conventional gene-delivery vectors.

See also: gene therapy, cloning vector

Chloroplast chromosome

Circular DNA found in the photosynthesizing organelle (chloroplast) of plants instead of the cell nucleus where most genetic material is located.

Chromomere

One of the serially aligned beads or granules of a eukaryotic chromosome, resulting from local coiling of a continuous DNA thread.

Chromosomal deletion

The loss of part of a chromosome's DNA.

Chromosomal inversion

Chromosome segments that have been turned 180 degrees. The gene sequence for the segment is reversed with respect to the rest of the chromosome.

Chromosome

The self-replicating genetic structure of cells containing the cellular DNA that bears in its nucleotide sequence the linear array of genes. In prokaryotes, chromosomal DNA is circular, and the entire genome is carried on one chromosome. Eukaryotic genomes consist of a number of chromosomes whose DNA is associated with different kinds of proteins.

Chromosome painting
> Attachment of certain fluorescent dyes to targeted parts of the chromosome. Used as a diagnositic for particular diseases, e.g. types of leukemia.

Chromosome region p
> A designation for the short arm of a chromosome.

Chromosome region q
> A designation for the long arm of a chromosome.

Clone
> An exact copy made of biological material such as a DNA segment (e.g., a gene or other region), a whole cell, or a complete organism.

Clone bank
> *See:* genomic library

Cloning
> Using specialized DNA technology to produce multiple, exact copies of a single gene or other segment of DNA to obtain enough material for further study. This process, used by researchers in the Human Genome Project, is referred to as cloning DNA. The resulting cloned (copied) collections of DNA molecules are called clone libraries. A second type of cloning exploits the natural process of cell division to make many copies of an entire cell. The genetic makeup of these cloned cells, called a cell line, is identical to the original cell. A third type of cloning produces complete, genetically identical animals such as the famous Scottish sheep, Dolly.
> *See also:* cloning vector

Cloning vector
> DNA molecule originating from a virus, a plasmid, or the cell of a higher organism into which another DNA fragment of appropriate size can be integrated without loss of the vector's capacity for self-replication; vectors introduce foreign DNA into host cells, where the DNA can be reproduced in large quantities. Examples are plasmids, cosmids, and yeast artificial chromosomes; vectors are often recombinant molecules containing DNA sequences from several sources.

Code
> *See:* genetic code

Codominance
> Situation in which two different alleles for a genetic trait are both expressed.
> *See also:* autosomal dominant, recessive gene

Codon
> *See:* genetic code

Coisogenic or congenic

Nearly identical strains of an organism; they vary at only a single locus.

Comparative genomics

The study of human genetics by comparisons with model organisms such as mice, the fruit fly, and the bacterium *E. coli*.

Complementary DNA (cDNA)

DNA that is synthesized in the laboratory from a messenger RNA template.

Complementary sequence

Nucleic acid base sequence that can form a double-stranded structure with another DNA fragment by following base-pairing rules (A pairs with T and C with G). The complementary sequence to GTAC for example, is CATG.

Complex trait

Trait that has a genetic component that does not follow strict Mendelian inheritance. May involve the interaction of two or more genes or gene-environment interactions.

See also: Mendelian inheritance, additive genetic effects

Computational biology

See: bioinformatics

Confidentiality

In genetics, the expectation that genetic material and the information gained from testing that material will not be available without the donor's consent.

Congenital

Any trait present at birth, whether the result of a genetic or nongenetic factor.

See also: birth defect

Conserved sequence

A base sequence in a DNA molecule (or an amino acid sequence in a protein) that has remained essentially unchanged throughout evolution.

Constitutive ablation

Gene expression that results in cell death.

Contig

Group of cloned (copied) pieces of DNA representing overlapping regions of a particular chromosome.

Contig map

A map depicting the relative order of a linked library of overlapping clones representing a complete chromosomal segment.

Cosmid

Artificially constructed cloning vector containing the cos gene of phage lambda. Cosmids can be packaged in lambda phage particles for infection into *E. coli*; this permits cloning of larger DNA fragments (up to 45kb) than can be introduced into bacterial hosts in plasmid vectors.

Crossing over
> The breaking during meiosis of one maternal and one paternal chromosome, the exchange of corresponding sections of DNA, and the rejoining of the chromosomes. This process can result in an exchange of alleles between chromosomes.
> *See also:* recombination

Cytogenetics
> The study of the physical appearance of chromosomes.
> *See also:* karyotype

Cytological band
> An area of the chromosome that stains differently from areas around it.
> *See also:* cytological map

Cytological map
> A type of chromosome map whereby genes are located on the basis of cytological findings obtained with the aid of chromosome mutations.

Cytoplasmic (uniparental) inheritance
> *See:* cytoplasmic trait

Cytoplasmic trait
> A genetic characteristic in which the genes are found outside the nucleus, in chloroplasts or mitochondria. Results in offspring inheriting genetic material from only one parent.

Cytosine (C)
> A nitrogenous base, one member of the base pair GC (guanine and cytosine) in DNA.
> *See also:* base pair, nucleotide

D

Data warehouse
> A collection of databases, data tables, and mechanisms to access the data on a single subject.

Deletion
> A loss of part of the DNA from a chromosome; can lead to a disease or abnormality.
> *See also:* chromosome, mutation

Deletion map
> A description of a specific chromosome that uses defined mutations—specific deleted areas in the genome—as 'biochemical signposts,' or markers for specific areas.

Deoxyribonucleotide

See: nucleotide

Deoxyribose

A type of sugar that is one component of DNA (deoxyribonucleic acid).

Diploid

A full set of genetic material consisting of paired chromosomes, one from each parental set. Most animal cells except the gametes have a diploid set of chromosomes. The diploid human genome has 46 chromosomes.

See also: haploid

Directed evolution

A laboratory process used on isolated molecules or microbes to cause mutations and identify subsequent adaptations to novel environments.

Directed mutagenesis

Alteration of DNA at a specific site and its reinsertion into an organism to study any effects of the change.

Directed sequencing

Successively sequencing DNA from adjacent stretches of chromosome.

Disease-associated genes

Alleles carrying particular DNA sequences associated with the presence of disease.

DNA (deoxyribonucleic acid)

The molecule that encodes genetic information. DNA is a double-stranded molecule held together by weak bonds between base pairs of nucleotides. The four nucleotides in DNA contain the bases adenine (A), guanine (G), cytosine (C), and thymine (T). In nature, base pairs form only between A and T and between G and C; thus the base sequence of each single strand can be deduced from that of its partner.

DNA bank

A service that stores DNA extracted from blood samples or other human tissue.

DNA probe

See: probe

DNA repair genes

Genes encoding proteins that correct errors in DNA sequencing.

DNA replication

The use of existing DNA as a template for the synthesis of new DNA strands. In humans and other eukaryotes, replication occurs in the cell nucleus.

DNA sequence

The relative order of base pairs, whether in a DNA fragment, gene, chromosome, or an entire genome.

See also: base sequence analysis

Domain

A discrete portion of a protein with its own function. The combination of domains in a single protein determines its overall function.

Dominant

An allele that is almost always expressed, even if only one copy is present.

See also: gene, genome

Double helix

The twisted-ladder shape that two linear strands of DNA assume when complementary nucleotides on opposing strands bond together.

Draft sequence

The sequence generated by the HGP as of June 2000 that, while incomplete, offers a virtual road map to an estimated 95% of all human genes. Draft sequence data are mostly in the form of 10,000 base pair-sized fragments whose approximate chromosomal locations are known.

See also: sequencing, finished DNA sequence, working draft DNA sequence.

E

Electrophoresis

A method of separating large molecules (such as DNA fragments or proteins) from a mixture of similar molecules. An electric current is passed through a medium containing the mixture, and each kind of molecule travels through the medium at a different rate, depending on its electrical charge and size. Agarose and acrylamide gels are the media commonly used for electrophoresis of proteins and nucleic acids.

Electroporation

A process using high-voltage current to make cell membranes permeable to allow the introduction of new DNA; commonly used in recombinant DNA technology.

See also: transfection

Embryonic stem (ES) cells

An embryonic cell that can replicate indefinitely, transform into other types of cells, and serve as a continuous source of new cells.

Endonuclease

See: restriction enzyme

Enzyme

> A protein that acts as a catalyst, speeding the rate at which a biochemical reaction proceeds but not altering the direction or nature of the reaction.

Epistasis

> One gene interfers with or prevents the expression of another gene located at a different locus.

Escherichia coli

> Common bacterium that has been studied intensively by geneticists because of its small genome size, normal lack of pathogenicity, and ease of growth in the laboratory.

Eugenics

> The study of improving a species by artificial selection; usually refers to the selective breeding of humans.

Eukaryote

> Cell or organism with membrane-bound, structurally discrete nucleus and other well-developed subcellular compartments. Eukaryotes include all organisms except viruses, bacteria, and bluegreen algae.
>
> *See also:* prokaryote, chromosome.

Evolutionarily conserved

> *See:* conserved sequence

Exogenous DNA

> DNA originating outside an organism that has been introduced into the organism.

Exon

> The protein-coding DNA sequence of a gene.
>
> *See also:* intron

Exonuclease

> An enzyme that cleaves nucleotides sequentially from free ends of a linear nucleic acid substrate.

Expressed gene

> *See:* gene expression

Expressed sequence tag (EST)

> A short strand of DNA that is a part of a cDNA molecule and can act as identifier of a gene. Used in locating and mapping genes.
>
> *See also:* cDNA, sequence tagged site

F

Filial generation (F1, F2)

> Each generation of offspring in a breeding program, designated F1, F2, etc.

Fingerprinting

In genetics, the identification of multiple specific alleles on a person's DNA to produce a unique identifier for that person.

See also: forensics

Finished DNA Sequence

High-quality, low error, gap-free DNA sequence of the human genome. Achieving this ultimate 2003 HGP goal requires additional sequencing to close gaps, reduce ambiguities, and allow for only a single error every 10,000 bases, the agreed-upon standard for HGP finished sequence.

See also: sequencing, draft sequence

Flow cytometry

Analysis of biological material by detection of the light-absorbing or fluorescing properties of cells or subcellular fractions (i.e., chromosomes) passing in a narrow stream through a laser beam. An absorbance or fluorescence profile of the sample is produced. Automated sorting devices, used to fractionate samples, sort successive droplets of the analyzed stream into different fractions depending on the fluorescence emitted by each droplet.

Flow karyotyping

Use of flow cytometry to analyze and separate chromosomes according to their DNA content.

Fluorescence in situ hybridization (FISH)

A physical mapping approach that uses fluorescein tags to detect hybridization of probes with metaphase chromosomes and with the less-condensed somatic interphase chromatin.

Forensics

The use of DNA for identification. Some examples of DNA use are to establish paternity in child support cases; establish the presence of a suspect at a crime scene, and identify accident victims.

Fraternal twin

Siblings born at the same time as the result of fertilization of two ova by two sperm. They share the same genetic relationship to each other as any other siblings.

See also: identical twin

Full gene sequence

The complete order of bases in a gene. This order determines which protein a gene will produce.

Functional genomics

The study of genes, their resulting proteins, and the role played by the proteins the body's biochemical processes.

G

Gamete
> Mature male or female reproductive cell (sperm or ovum) with a haploid set of chromosomes (23 for humans).

GC-rich area
> Many DNA sequences carry long stretches of repeated G and C which often indicate a gene-rich region.

Gel electrophoresis
> *See:* electrophoresis

Gene
> The fundamental physical and functional unit of heredity. A gene is an ordered sequence of nucleotides located in a particular position on a particular chromosome that encodes a specific functional product (i.e., a protein or RNA molecule).
> *See also:* gene expression

Gene amplification
> Repeated copying of a piece of DNA; a characteristic of tumor cells.
> *See also:* gene, oncogene

Gene chip technology
> Development of cDNA microarrays from a large number of genes. Used to monitor and measure changes in gene expression for each gene represented on the chip.

Gene expression
> The process by which a gene's coded information is converted into the structures present and operating in the cell. Expressed genes include those that are transcribed into mRNA and then translated into protein and those that are transcribed into RNA but not translated into protein (e.g., transfer and ribosomal RNAs).

Gene family
> Group of closely related genes that make similar products.

Gene library
> *See:* genomic library

Gene mapping
> Determination of the relative positions of genes on a DNA molecule (chromosome or plasmid) and of the distance, in linkage units or physical units, between them.

Gene pool
> All the variations of genes in a species.
> *See also:* allele, gene, polymorphism

Gene prediction
Predictions of possible genes made by a computer program based on how well a stretch of DNA sequence matches known gene sequences

Gene product
The biochemical material, either RNA or protein, resulting from expression of a gene. The amount of gene product is used to measure how active a gene is; abnormal amounts can be correlated with disease-causing alleles.

Gene testing
See: genetic testing, genetic screening

Gene therapy
An experimental procedure aimed at replacing, manipulating, or supplementing nonfunctional or misfunctioning genes with healthy genes.
See also: gene, inherit, somatic cell gene therapy, germ line gene therapy

Gene transfer
Incorporation of new DNA into and organism's cells, usually by a vector such as a modified virus. Used in gene therapy.
See also: mutation, gene therapy, vector

Genetic code
The sequence of nucleotides, coded in triplets (codons) along the mRNA, that determines the sequence of amino acids in protein synthesis. A gene's DNA sequence can be used to predict the mRNA sequence, and the genetic code can in turn be used to predict the amino acid sequence.

Genetic counseling
Provides patients and their families with education and information about genetic-related conditions and helps them make informed decisions.

Genetic discrimination
Prejudice against those who have or are likely to develop an inherited disorder.

Genetic engineering
Altering the genetic material of cells or organisms to enable them to make new substances or perform new functions.

Genetic engineering technology
See: recombinant DNA technology

Genetic illness
Sickness, physical disability, or other disorder resulting from the inheritance of one or more deleterious alleles.

Genetic informatics
See: bioinformatics

Genetic map
See: linkage map

Genetic marker

A gene or other identifiable portion of DNA whose inheritance can be followed.

See also: chromosome, DNA, gene, inherit

Genetic material

See: genome

Genetic mosaic

An organism in which different cells contain different genetic sequence. This can be the result of a mutation during development or fusion of embryos at an early developmental stage.

Genetic polymorphism

Difference in DNA sequence among individuals, groups, or populations (e.g., genes for blue eyes versus brown eyes).

Genetic predisposition

Susceptibility to a genetic disease. May or may not result in actual development of the disease.

Genetic screening

Testing a group of people to identify individuals at high risk of having or passing on a specific genetic disorder.

Genetic testing

Analyzing an individual's genetic material to determine predisposition to a particular health condition or to confirm a diagnosis of genetic disease.

Genetics

The study of inheritance patterns of specific traits.

Genome

All the genetic material in the chromosomes of a particular organism; its size is generally given as its total number of base pairs.

Genome project

Research and technology-development effort aimed at mapping and sequencing the genome of human beings and certain model organisms.

See also: Human Genome Initiative

Genomic library

A collection of clones made from a set of randomly generated overlapping DNA fragments that represent the entire genome of an organism.

See also: library, arrayed library

Genomic sequence

See: DNA

Genomics

The study of genes and their function.

Genotype
> The genetic constitution of an organism, as distinguished from its physical appearance (its phenotype).

Germ cell
> Sperm and egg cells and their precursors. Germ cells are haploid and have only one set of chromosomes (23 in all), while all other cells have two copies (46 in all).

Germ line
> The continuation of a set of genetic information from one generation to the next.
> *See also:* inherit

Germ line gene therapy
> An experimental process of inserting genes into germ cells or fertilized eggs to cause a genetic change that can be passed on to offspring. May be used to alleviate effects associated with a genetic disease.
> *See also:* genomics, somatic cell gene therapy.

Germ line genetic mutation
> *See:* mutation

Guanine (G)
> A nitrogenous base, one member of the base pair GC (guanine and cytosine) in DNA.
> *See also:* base pair, nucleotide

Gyandromorph
> Organisms that have both male and female cells and therefore express both male and female characteristics.

H

Haploid
> A single set of chromosomes (half the full set of genetic material) present in the egg and sperm cells of animals and in the egg and pollen cells of plants. Human beings have 23 chromosomes in their reproductive cells.
> *See also:* diploid

Haplotype
> A way of denoting the collective genotype of a number of closely linked loci on a chromosome.

Hemizygous
> Having only one copy of a particular gene. For example, in humans, males are hemizygous for genes found on the Y chromosome.

Hereditary cancer

Cancer that occurs due to the inheritance of an altered gene within a family.
See also: sporadic cancer

Heterozygosity

The presence of different alleles at one or more loci on homologous chromosomes.

Heterozygote

See: heterozygosity

Highly conserved sequence

DNA sequence that is very similar across several different types of organisms.
See also: gene, mutation

High-throughput sequencing

A fast method of determining the order of bases in DNA.
See also: sequencing

Homeobox

A short stretch of nucleotides whose base sequence is virtually identical in all the genes that contain it. Homeoboxes have been found in many organisms from fruit flies to human beings. In the fruit fly, a homeobox appears to determine when particular groups of genes are expressed during development.

Homolog

A member of a chromosome pair in diploid organisms or a gene that has the same origin and functions in two or more species.

Homologous chromosome

Chromosome containing the same linear gene sequences as another, each derived from one parent.

Homologous recombination

Swapping of DNA fragments between paired chromosomes.

Homology

Similarity in DNA or protein sequences between individuals of the same species or among different species.

Homozygote

An organism that has two identical alleles of a gene.
See also: heterozygote

Homozygous

See: homozygote

Human artificial chromosome (HAC)

A vector used to hold large DNA fragments.
See also: chromosome, DNA

Human gene therapy
> *See:* gene therapy

Human Genome Initiative
> Collective name for several projects begun in 1986 by DOE to create an ordered set of DNA segments from known chromosomal locations, develop new computational methods for analyzing genetic map and DNA sequence data, and develop new techniques and instruments for detecting and analyzing DNA. This DOE initiative is now known as the Human Genome Program. The joint national effort, led by DOE and NIH, is known as the Human Genome Project.

Human Genome Project (HGP)
> Formerly titled Human Genome Initiative.
> *See also:* Human Genome Initiative

Hybrid
> The offspring of genetically different parents.
> *See also:* heterozygote

Hybridization
> The process of joining two complementary strands of DNA or one each of DNA and RNA to form a double-stranded molecule.

I

Identical twin
> Twins produced by the division of a single zygote; both have identical genotypes.
> *See also:* fraternal twin

Immunotherapy
> Using the immune system to treat disease, for example, in the development of vaccines. May also refer to the therapy of diseases caused by the immune system.
> *See also:* cancer

Imprinting
> A phenomenon in which the disease phenotype depends on which parent passed on the disease gene. For instance, both Prader-Willi and Angelman syndromes are inherited when the same part of chromosome 15 is missing. When the father's complement of 15 is missing, the child has Prader-Willi, but when the mother's complement of 15 is missing, the child has Angelman syndrome.

In situ hybridization

Use of a DNA or RNA probe to detect the presence of the complementary DNA sequence in cloned bacterial or cultured eukaryotic cells.

In vitro

Studies performed outside a living organism such as in a laboratory.

In vivo

Studies carried out in living organisms.

Independent assortment

During meiosis each of the two copies of a gene is distributed to the germ cells independently of the distribution of other genes.

See also: linkage

Informatics

See: bioinformatics

Informed consent

An individual willingly agrees to participate in an activity after first being advised of the risks and benefits.

See also: privacy

Inherit

In genetics, to receive genetic material from parents through biological processes.

Inherited

See: inherit

Insertion

A chromosome abnormality in which a piece of DNA is incorporated into a gene and thereby disrupts the gene's normal function.

See also: chromosome, DNA, gene, mutation

Insertional mutation

See: insertion

Intellectual property rights

Patents, copyrights, and trademarks.

See also: patent

Interference

One crossover event inhibits the chances of another crossover event. Also known as positive interference. Negative interference increases the chance of a second crossover.

See also: crossing over

Interphase

The period in the cell cycle when DNA is replicated in the nucleus; followed by mitosis.

Intron
> DNA sequence that interrupts the protein-coding sequence of a gene; an intron is transcribed into RNA but is cut out of the message before it is translated into protein.
> *See also:* exon

Isoenzyme
> An enzyme performing the same function as another enzyme but having a different set of amino acids. The two enzymes may function at different speeds.

J

Junk DNA
> Stretches of DNA that do not code for genes; most of the genome consists of so-called junk DNA which may have regulatory and other functions. Also called non-coding DNA.

K

Karyotype
> A photomicrograph of an individual's chromosomes arranged in a standard format showing the number, size, and shape of each chromosome type; used in low-resolution physical mapping to correlate gross chromosomal abnormalities with the characteristics of specific diseases.

Kilobase (kb)
> Unit of length for DNA fragments equal to 1000 nucleotides.

Knockout
> Deactivation of specific genes; used in laboratory organisms to study gene function.
> *See also:* gene, locus, model organisms

L

Library
> An unordered collection of clones (i.e., cloned DNA from a particular organism) whose relationship to each other can be established by physical mapping.
> *See also:* genomic library, arrayed library

Linkage
> The proximity of two or more markers (e.g., genes, RFLP markers) on a chromosome; the closer the markers, the lower the probability that they will be separated during DNA repair or replication processes (binary fission in prokaryotes, mitosis or meiosis in eukaryotes), and hence the greater the probability that they will be inherited together.

Linkage disequilibrium
> Where alleles occur together more often than can be accounted for by chance. Indicates that the two alleles are physically close on the DNA strand.
>
> *See also:* Mendelian inheritance

Linkage map
> A map of the relative positions of genetic loci on a chromosome, determined on the basis of how often the loci are inherited together. Distance is measured in centimorgans (cM).

Localize
> Determination of the original position (locus) of a gene or other marker on a chromosome.

Locus (pl. loci)
> The position on a chromosome of a gene or other chromosome marker; also, the DNA at that position. The use of locus is sometimes restricted to mean expressed DNA regions.
>
> *See also:* gene expression

Long-Range Restriction Mapping
> Restriction enzymes are proteins that cut DNA at precise locations. Restriction maps depict the chromosomal positions of restriction-enzyme cutting sites. These are used as biochemical "signposts," or markers of specific areas along the chromosomes. The map will detail the positions where the DNA molecule is cut by particular restriction enzymes.

M

Macrorestriction map
> Map depicting the order of and distance between sites at which restriction enzymes cleave chromosomes.

Mapping
> *See:* gene mapping, linkage map, physical map

Mapping population
> The group of related organisms used in constructing a genetic map.

Marker
> *See:* genetic marker

Mass spectrometry
> An instrument used to identify chemicals in a substance by their mass and charge.

Megabase (Mb)
> Unit of length for DNA fragments equal to 1 million nucleotides and roughly equal to 1 cM.
> *See also:* centimorgan

Meiosis
> The process of two consecutive cell divisions in the diploid progenitors of sex cells. Meiosis results in four rather than two daughter cells, each with a haploid set of chromosomes.
> *See also:* mitosis

Mendelian inheritance
> One method in which genetic traits are passed from parents to offspring. Named for Gregor Mendel, who first studied and recognized the existence of genes and this method of inheritance.
> *See also:* autosomal dominant, recessive gene, sex-linked

Messenger RNA (mRNA)
> RNA that serves as a template for protein synthesis.
> *See also:* genetic code

Metaphase
> A stage in mitosis or meiosis during which the chromosomes are aligned along the equatorial plane of the cell.

Microarray
> Sets of miniaturized chemical reaction areas that may also be used to test DNA fragments, antibodies, or proteins.

Microbial genetics
> The study of genes and gene function in bacteria, archaea, and other microorganisms. Often used in research in the fields of bioremediation, alternative energy, and disease prevention.
> *See also:* model organisms, biotechnology, bioremediation

Microinjection
> A technique for introducing a solution of DNA into a cell using a fine microcapillary pipet.

Micronuclei
> Chromosome fragments that are not incorporated into the nucleus at cell division.

Mitochondrial DNA

The genetic material found in mitochondria, the organelles that generate energy for the cell. Not inherited in the same fashion as nucleic DNA.

See also: cell, DNA, genome, nucleus

Mitosis

The process of nuclear division in cells that produces daughter cells that are genetically identical to each other and to the parent cell.

See also: meiosis

Model organisms

A laboratory animal or other organism useful for research.

Modeling

The use of statistical analysis, computer analysis, or model organisms to predict outcomes of research.

Molecular biology

The study of the structure, function, and makeup of biologically important molecules.

Molecular farming

The development of transgenic animals to produce human proteins for medical use.

Molecular genetics

The study of macromolecules important in biological inheritance.

Molecular medicine

The treatment of injury or disease at the molecular level. Examples include the use of DNA-based diagnostic tests or medicine derived from DNA sequence information.

Monogenic disorder

A disorder caused by mutation of a single gene.

See also: mutation, polygenic disorder

Monogenic inheritance

See: monogenic disorder

Monosomy

Possessing only one copy of a particular chromosome instead of the normal two copies.

See also: cell, chromosome, gene expression, trisomy

Morbid map

A diagram showing the chromosomal location of genes associated with disease.

Mouse model

See: model organisms

Multifactorial or multigenic disorder
> *See:* polygenic disorder

Multiplexing
> A laboratory approach that performs multiple sets of reactions in parallel (simultaneously); greatly increasing speed and throughput.

Murine
> Organism in the genus Mus. A rat or mouse.

Mutagen
> An agent that causes a permanent genetic change in a cell. Does not include changes occurring during normal genetic recombination.

Mutagenicity
> The capacity of a chemical or physical agent to cause permanent genetic alterations.
> *See also:* somatic cell genetic mutation

Mutation
> Any heritable change in DNA sequence.
> *See also:* polymorphism

N

Nitrogenous base
> A nitrogen-containing molecule having the chemical properties of a base. DNA contains the nitrogenous bases adenine (A), guanine (G), cytosine (C), and thymine (T).
> *See also:* DNA

Northern blot
> A gel-based laboratory procedure that locates mRNA sequences on a gel that are complementary to a piece of DNA used as a probe.
> *See also:* DNA, library

Nuclear transfer
> A laboratory procedure in which a cell's nucleus is removed and placed into an oocyte with its own nucleus removed so the genetic information from the donor nucleus controls the resulting cell. Such cells can be induced to form embryos. This process was used to create the cloned sheep "Dolly".
> *See also:* cloning

Nucleic acid
> A large molecule composed of nucleotide subunits.
> *See also:* DNA

Nucleolar organizing region
> A part of the chromosome containing rRNA genes.

Nucleotide

A subunit of DNA or RNA consisting of a nitrogenous base (adenine, guanine, thymine, or cytosine in DNA; adenine, guanine, uracil, or cytosine in RNA), a phosphate molecule, and a sugar molecule (deoxyribose in DNA and ribose in RNA). Thousands of nucleotides are linked to form a DNA or RNA molecule.

See also: DNA, base pair, RNA

Nucleus

The cellular organelle in eukaryotes that contains most of the genetic material.

O

Oligo

See: oligonucleotide

Oligogenic

A phenotypic trait produced by two or more genes working together.

See also: polygenic disorder

Oligonucleotide

A molecule usually composed of 25 or fewer nucleotides; used as a DNA synthesis primer.

See also: nucleotide

Oncogene

A gene, one or more forms of which is associated with cancer. Many oncogenes are involved, directly or indirectly, in controlling the rate of cell growth.

Open reading frame (ORF)

The sequence of DNA or RNA located between the start-code sequence (initiation codon) and the stop-code sequence (termination codon).

Operon

A set of genes transcribed under the control of an operator gene.

Overlapping clones

See: genomic library

P

P1-derived artificial chromosome (PAC)

One type of vector used to clone DNA fragments (100-to 300-kb insert size; average, 150 kb) in *Escherichia coli* cells. Based on bacteriophage (a virus) P1 genome.

See also: cloning vector

Patent

In genetics, conferring the right or title to genes, gene variations, or identifiable portions of sequenced genetic material to an individual or organization. *See also:* gene

Pedigree

A family tree diagram that shows how a particular genetic trait or disease has been inherited. *See also:* inherit

Penetrance

The probability of a gene or genetic trait being expressed. "Complete" penetrance means the gene or genes for a trait are expressed in all the population who have the genes. "Incomplete" penetrance means the genetic trait is expressed in only part of the population. The percent penetrance also may change with the age range of the population.

Peptide

Two or more amino acids joined by a bond called a "peptide bond." *See also:* polypeptide

Phage

A virus for which the natural host is a bacterial cell.

Pharmacogenomics

The study of the interaction of an individual's genetic makeup and response to a drug.

Phenocopy

A trait not caused by inheritance of a gene but appears to be identical to a genetic trait.

Phenotype

The physical characteristics of an organism or the presence of a disease that may or may not be genetic. *See also:* genotype

Physical map

A map of the locations of identifiable landmarks on DNA (e.g., restriction-enzyme cutting sites, genes), regardless of inheritance. Distance is measured in base pairs. For the human genome, the lowest-resolution physical map is the banding patterns on the 24 different chromosomes; the highest-resolution map is the complete nucleotide sequence of the chromosomes.

Plasmid

Autonomously replicating extra-chromosomal circular DNA molecules, distinct from the normal bacterial genome and nonessential for cell survival under nonselective conditions. Some plasmids are capable of integrating into the host genome. A number of artificially constructed plasmids are used as cloning vectors.

Pleiotropy

One gene that causes many different physical traits such as multiple disease symptoms.

Pluripotency

The potential of a cell to develop into more than one type of mature cell, depending on environment.

Polygenic disorder

Genetic disorder resulting from the combined action of alleles of more than one gene (e.g., heart disease, diabetes, and some cancers). Although such disorders are inherited, they depend on the simultaneous presence of several alleles; thus the hereditary patterns usually are more complex than those of single-gene disorders.

See also: single-gene disorder

Polymerase chain reaction (PCR)

A method for amplifying a DNA base sequence using a heat-stable polymerase and two 20-base primers, one complementary to the (+) strand at one end of the sequence to be amplified and one complementary to the (-) strand at the other end. Because the newly synthesized DNA strands can subsequently serve as additional templates for the same primer sequences, successive rounds of primer annealing, strand elongation, and dissociation produce rapid and highly specific amplification of the desired sequence. PCR also can be used to detect the existence of the defined sequence in a DNA sample.

Polymerase, DNA or RNA

Enzyme that catalyzes the synthesis of nucleic acids on preexisting nucleic acid templates, assembling RNA from ribonucleotides or DNA from deoxyribonucleotides.

Polymorphism

Difference in DNA sequence among individuals that may underlie differences in health. Genetic variations occurring in more than 1% of a population would be considered useful polymorphisms for genetic linkage analysis.

See also: mutation

Polypeptide

A protein or part of a protein made of a chain of amino acids joined by a peptide bond.

Population genetics

The study of variation in genes among a group of individuals.

Positional cloning

A technique used to identify genes, usually those that are associated with diseases, based on their location on a chromosome.

Premature chromosome condensation (PCC)

A method of studying chromosomes in the interphase stage of the cell cycle.

Primer

Short preexisting polynucleotide chain to which new deoxyribonucleotides can be added by DNA polymerase.

Privacy

In genetics, the right of people to restrict access to their genetic information.

Probe

Single-stranded DNA or RNA molecules of specific base sequence, labeled either radioactively or immunologically, that are used to detect the complementary base sequence by hybridization.

Prokaryote

Cell or organism lacking a membrane-bound, structurally discrete nucleus and other subcellular compartments. Bacteria are examples of prokaryotes. *See also:* chromosome, eukaryote

Promoter

A DNA site to which RNA polymerase will bind and initiate transcription.

Pronucleus

The nucleus of a sperm or egg prior to fertilization. *See also:* nucleus, transgenic

Protein

A large molecule composed of one or more chains of amino acids in a specific order; the order is determined by the base sequence of nucleotides in the gene that codes for the protein. Proteins are required for the structure, function, and regulation of the body's cells, tissues, and organs; and each protein has unique functions. Examples are hormones, enzymes, and antibodies.

Proteome

Proteins expressed by a cell or organ at a particular time and under specific conditions.

Proteomics

The study of the full set of proteins encoded by a genome.

Pseudogene

A sequence of DNA similar to a gene but nonfunctional; probably the remnant of a once-functional gene that accumulated mutations.

Purine

A nitrogen-containing, double-ring, basic compound that occurs in nucleic acids. The purines in DNA and RNA are adenine and guanine.

See also: base pair

Pyrimidine

A nitrogen-containing, single-ring, basic compound that occurs in nucleic acids. The pyrimidines in DNA are cytosine and thymine; in RNA, cytosine and uracil.

See also: base pair

R

Radiation hybrid

A hybrid cell containing small fragments of irradiated human chromosomes. Maps of irradiation sites on chromosomes for the human, rat, mouse, and other genomes provide important markers, allowing the construction of very precise STS maps indispensable to studying multifactorial diseases.

See also: sequence tagged site

Rare-cutter enzyme

See: restriction-enzyme cutting site

Recessive gene

A gene which will be expressed only if there are 2 identical copies or, for a male, if one copy is present on the X chromosome.

Reciprocal translocation

When a pair of chromosomes exchange exactly the same length and area of DNA. Results in a shuffling of genes.

Recombinant clone

Clone containing recombinant DNA molecules.

See also: recombinant DNA technology

Recombinant DNA molecules

A combination of DNA molecules of different origin that are joined using recombinant DNA technologies.

Recombinant DNA technology

Procedure used to join together DNA segments in a cell-free system (an environment outside a cell or organism). Under appropriate conditions, a recombinant DNA molecule can enter a cell and replicate there, either autonomously or after it has become integrated into a cellular chromosome.

Recombination

The process by which progeny derive a combination of genes different from that of either parent. In higher organisms, this can occur by crossing over.

See also: crossing over, mutation

Regulatory region or sequence

A DNA base sequence that controls gene expression.

Repetitive DNA

Sequences of varying lengths that occur in multiple copies in the genome; it represents much of the human genome.

Reporter gene

See: marker

Resolution

Degree of molecular detail on a physical map of DNA, ranging from low to high.

Restriction enzyme, endonuclease

A protein that recognizes specific, short nucleotide sequences and cuts DNA at those sites. Bacteria contain over 400 such enzymes that recognize and cut more than 100 different DNA sequences.

See also: restriction enzyme cutting site

Restriction fragment length polymorphism (RFLP)

Variation between individuals in DNA fragment sizes cut by specific restriction enzymes; polymorphic sequences that result in RFLPs are used as markers on both physical maps and genetic linkage maps. RFLPs usually are caused by mutation at a cutting site.

See also: marker, polymorphism

Restriction-enzyme cutting site

A specific nucleotide sequence of DNA at which a particular restriction enzyme cuts the DNA. Some sites occur frequently in DNA (e.g., every several hundred base pairs); others much less frequently (rare-cutter; e.g., every 10,000 base pairs).

Retroviral infection

The presence of retroviral vectors, such as some viruses, which use their recombinant DNA to insert their genetic material into the chromosomes of the host's cells. The virus is then propogated by the host cell.

Reverse transcriptase

An enzyme used by retroviruses to form a complementary DNA sequence (cDNA) from their RNA. The resulting DNA is then inserted into the chromosome of the host cell.

Ribonucleotide

See: nucleotide

Ribose

The five-carbon sugar that serves as a component of RNA.

See also: ribonucleic acid, deoxyribose

Ribosomal RNA (rRNA)

A class of RNA found in the ribosomes of cells.

Ribosomes

Small cellular components composed of specialized ribosomal RNA and protein; site of protein synthesis.

See also: RNA

Risk communication

In genetics, a process in which a genetic counselor or other medical professional interprets genetic test results and advises patients of the consequences for them and their offspring.

RNA (Ribonucleic acid)

A chemical found in the nucleus and cytoplasm of cells; it plays an important role in protein synthesis and other chemical activities of the cell. The structure of RNA is similar to that of DNA. There are several classes of RNA molecules, including messenger RNA, transfer RNA, ribosomal RNA, and other small RNAs, each serving a different purpose.

S

Sanger sequencing

A widely used method of determining the order of bases in DNA.

See also: sequencing, shotgun sequencing

Satellite

A chromosomal segment that branches off from the rest of the chromosome but is still connected by a thin filament or stalk.

Scaffold

In genomic mapping, a series of contigs that are in the right order but not necessarily connected in one continuous stretch of sequence.

Segregation

The normal biological process whereby the two pieces of a chromosome pair are separated during meiosis and randomly distributed to the germ cells.

Sequence

See: base sequence

Sequence assembly

A process whereby the order of multiple sequenced DNA fragments is determined.

Sequence tagged site (STS)

Short (200 to 500 base pairs) DNA sequence that has a single occurrence in the human genome and whose location and base sequence are known. Detectable by polymerase chain reaction, STSs are useful for localizing and orienting the mapping and sequence data reported from many different laboratories and serve as landmarks on the developing physical map of the human genome. Expressed sequence tags (ESTs) are STSs derived from cDNAs.

Sequencing

Determination of the order of nucleotides (base sequences) in a DNA or RNA molecule or the order of amino acids in a protein.

Sequencing technology

The instrumentation and procedures used to determine the order of nucleotides in DNA.

Sex chromosome

The X or Y chromosome in human beings that determines the sex of an individual. Females have two X chromosomes in diploid cells; males have an X and a Y chromosome. The sex chromosomes comprise the 23rd chromosome pair in a karyotype.

See also: autosome

Sex-linked

Traits or diseases associated with the X or Y chromosome; generally seen in males.

See also: gene, mutation, sex chromosome

Shotgun method

Sequencing method that involves randomly sequenced cloned pieces of the genome, with no foreknowledge of where the piece originally came from. This can be contrasted with "directed" strategies, in which pieces of DNA from known chromosomal locations are sequenced. Because there are advantages to both strategies, researchers use both random (or shotgun) and directed strategies in combination to sequence the human genome.

See also: library, genomic library

Single nucleotide polymorphism (SNP)

DNA sequence variations that occur when a single nucleotide (A, T, C, or G) in the genome sequence is altered.

See also: mutation, polymorphism, single-gene disorder

Single-gene disorder

Hereditary disorder caused by a mutant allele of a single gene (e.g., Duchenne muscular dystrophy, retinoblastoma, sickle cell disease).

See also: <u>polygenic disorders</u>

Somatic cell

Any cell in the body except gametes and their precursors.

See also: <u>gamete</u>

Somatic cell gene therapy

Incorporating new genetic material into cells for therapeutic purposes. The new genetic material cannot be passed to offspring.

See also: <u>gene therapy</u>

Somatic cell genetic mutation

A change in the genetic structure that is neither inherited nor passed to offspring. Also called acquired mutations.

See also: <u>germ line genetic mutation</u>

Southern blotting

Transfer by absorption of DNA fragments separated in electrophoretic gels to membrane filters for detection of specific base sequences by radio-labeled complementary probes.

Spectral karyotype (SKY)

A graphic of all an organism's chromosomes, each labeled with a different color. Useful for identifying chromosomal abnormalities.

See also: <u>chromosome</u>

Splice site

Location in the DNA sequence where RNA removes the noncoding areas to form a continuous gene transcript for translation into a protein.

Sporadic cancer

Cancer that occurs randomly and is not inherited from parents. Caused by DNA changes in one cell that grows and divides, spreading throughout the body.

See also: <u>hereditary cancer</u>

Stem cell

Undifferentiated, primitive cells in the bone marrow that have the ability both to multiply and to differentiate into specific blood cells.

Structural genomics

The effort to determine the 3D structures of large numbers of proteins using both experimental techniques and computer simulation

Substitution

In genetics, a type of mutation due to replacement of one nucleotide in a DNA sequence by another nucleotide or replacement of one amino acid in a protein by another amino acid.

See also: mutation

Suppressor gene

A gene that can suppress the action of another gene.

Syndrome

The group or recognizable pattern of symptoms or abnormalities that indicate a particular trait or disease.

Syngeneic

Genetically identical members of the same species.

Synteny

Genes occurring in the same order on chromosomes of different species.

See also: linkage, conserved sequence

T

Tandem repeat sequences

Multiple copies of the same base sequence on a chromosome; used as markers in physical mapping.

See also: physical map

Targeted mutagenesis

Deliberate change in the genetic structure directed at a specific site on the chromosome. Used in research to determine the targeted region's function.

See also: mutation, polymorphism

Technology transfer

The process of transferring scientific findings from research laboratories to the commercial sector.

Telomerase

The enzyme that directs the replication of telomeres.

Telomere

The end of a chromosome. This specialized structure is involved in the replication and stability of linear DNA molecules.

See also: DNA replication

Teratogenic

Substances such as chemicals or radiation that cause abnormal development of a embryo.

See also: mutatgen

Thymine (T)

A nitrogenous base, one member of the base pair AT (adenine-thymine). *See also:* base pair, nucleotide

Toxicogenomics

The study of how genomes respond to environmental stressors or toxicants. Combines genome-wide mRNA expression profiling with protein expression patterns using bioinformatics to understand the role of gene-environment interactions in disease and dysfunction.

Transcription

The synthesis of an RNA copy from a sequence of DNA (a gene); the first step in gene expression. *See also:* translation

Transcription factor

A protein that binds to regulatory regions and helps control gene expression.

Transcriptome

The full complement of activated genes, mRNAs, or transcripts in a particular tissue at a particular time

Transfection

The introduction of foreign DNA into a host cell. *See also:* cloning vector, gene therapy

Transfer RNA (tRNA)

A class of RNA having structures with triplet nucleotide sequences that are complementary to the triplet nucleotide coding sequences of mRNA. The role of tRNAs in protein synthesis is to bond with amino acids and transfer them to the ribosomes, where proteins are assembled according to the genetic code carried by mRNA.

Transformation

A process by which the genetic material carried by an individual cell is altered by incorporation of exogenous DNA into its genome.

Transgenic

An experimentally produced organism in which DNA has been artificially introduced and incorporated into the organism's germ line. *See also:* cell, DNA, gene, nucleus, germ line

Translation

The process in which the genetic code carried by mRNA directs the synthesis of proteins from amino acids. *See also:* transcription

Translocation
> A mutation in which a large segment of one chromosome breaks off and attaches to another chromosome.
> *See also:* <u>mutation</u>

Transposable element
> A class of DNA sequences that can move from one chromosomal site to another.

Trisomy
> Possessing three copies of a particular chromosome instead of the normal two copies.
> *See also:* <u>cell, gene, gene expression, chromosome</u>

U

Uracil
> A nitrogenous base normally found in RNA but not DNA; uracil is capable of forming a base pair with adenine.
> *See also:* <u>base pair, nucleotide</u>

V

Vector
> *See:* <u>cloning vector</u>

Virus
> A noncellular biological entity that can reproduce only within a host cell. Viruses consist of nucleic acid covered by protein; some animal viruses are also surrounded by membrane. Inside the infected cell, the virus uses the synthetic capability of the host to produce progeny virus.
> *See also:* <u>cloning vector</u>

W

Western blot
> A technique used to identify and locate proteins based on their ability to bind to specific antibodies.
> *See also:* <u>DNA, Northern blot, protein, RNA, Southern blotting</u>

Wild type
> The form of an organism that occurs most frequently in nature.

Working Draft DNA Sequence
> *See:* <u>Draft DNA Sequence</u>

X

X chromosome
>One of the two sex chromosomes, X and Y.
>*See also:* Y chromosome, sex chromosome

Xenograft
>Tissue or organs from an individual of one species transplanted into or grafted onto an organism of another species, genus, or family. A common example is the use of pig heart valves in humans.

Y

Y chromosome
>One of the two sex chromosomes, X and Y.
>*See also:* X chromosome, sex chromosome

Yeast artificial chromosome (YAC)
>Constructed from yeast DNA, it is a vector used to clone large DNA fragments.
>*See also:* cloning vector, cosmid

Z

Zinc-finger protein
>A secondary feature of some proteins containing a zinc atom; a DNA-binding protein.
>Updated 12-Oct-02

The online presentation of this publication is a special feature of the Human Genome Project Information Web site.

This document may be cited in the following style:
Human Genome Program, U.S. Department of Energy, *Genomics and Its Impact on Medicine and Society: A 2001 Primer*, 2001.

For printed copies, please contact Laura Yust at Oak Ridge National Laboratory. Send questions or comments to the author, Denise K. Casey. Site designed by Marissa Mills.

Appendix B

Ethnic Genealogy Web Sites
(Usually, there are several genealogy sites on the Web for each ethnic group.)
Acadian/Cajun: & French Canadian: http://www.acadian.org/tidbits.html
Afghanistan Genealogy: http://www.kindredtrails.com/afghanistan.html
African-American: http://www.cyndislist.com/african.htm
African Royalty Genealogy: http://www.uq.net.au/~zzhsoszy/
Albanian Research List: http://feefhs.org/al/alrl.html
Armenian Genealogical Society: http://feefhs.org/am/frg-amgs.html
Asia and the Pacific: http://www.cyndislist.com/asia.htm
Austria-Hungary Empire: http://feefhs.org/ah/indexah.html
Baltic-Russian Information Center: http://feefhs.org/blitz/frgblitz.html
Belarusian—Association of the Belarusian Nobility: http://feefhs.org/by/frg-zbs.html
Bukovina Genealogy: http://feefhs.org/bukovina/bukovina.html
Carpatho-Rusyn Knowledge Base: http://feefhs.org/rusyn/frg-crkb.html
Chinese Genealogy: http://www.chineseroots.com.
Croatia Genealogy Cross Index: http://feefhs.org/cro/indexcro.html
Czechoslovak Genealogical Society Int'l, Inc.: http://feefhs.org/czs/cgsi/frg-cgsi.html
Eastern Europe: http://www.cyndislist.com/easteuro.htm
Eastern European Genealogical Society, Inc.: http://feefhs.org/ca/frg-eegs.html
Eastern Europe Ethnic, Religious, and National Index with Home Pages
includes the FEEFHS Resource Guide that lists organizations associated with
FEEFHS from 14 Countries. It also includes Finnish and Armenian genealogy
resources: http://feefhs.org/ethnic.html
Ethnic, Religious, and National Index 14 countries:
http://feefhs.org/ethnic.html
(Finland) Genealogical Society of Finland: http://www.genealogia.fi/indexe.htm
Finnish Genealogy Group: http://feefhs.org/misc/frgfinmn.html
Galicia Jewish SIG: http://feefhs.org/jsig/frg-gsig.html
German Genealogical Digest: http://feefhs.org/pub/frg-ggdp.html
Greek Genealogy Sources on the Internet: http://www-
personal.umich.edu/~cgaunt/greece.html
Genealogy Societies Online List: http://www.daddezio.com/catalog/grkndx04.html
German Research Association: http://feefhs.org/gra/frg-gra.html

Greek Genealogy (Hellenes-Diaspora Greek Genealogy):
http://www.geocities.com/SouthBeach/Cove/4537/
Greek Genealogy Home Page: http://www.daddezio.com/grekgen.html
Greek Genealogy Articles: http://www.daddezio.com/catalog/grkndx01.html
India Genealogy: http://genforum.genealogy.com/india/
India Family Histories:
http://www.mycinnamontoast.com/perl/results.cgi?region=79&sort=n
India-Anglo-Indian/Europeans in India genealogy:
http://members.ozemail.com.au/~clday/
Irish Travellers: http://www.pitt.edu/~alkst3/Traveller.html
Japanese Genealogy: http://www.rootsweb.com/~jpnwgw/
Jewish Genealogy: http://www.jewishgen.org/infofiles/
Latvian Jewish Genealogy Page: http://feefhs.org/jsig/frg-lsig.html
Lebanese Genealogy: http://www.rootsweb.com/~lbnwgw/
Lithuanian American Genealogy Society: http://feefhs.org/frg-lags.html
Melungeon: http://www.geocities.com/Paris/5121/melungeon.htm
Mennonite Heritage Center: http://feefhs.org/men/frg-mhc.html
Middle East Genealogy: http://www.rootsweb.com/~mdeastgw/index.html
Middle East Genealogy by country:
http://www.rootsweb.com/~mdeastgw/index.html#country
Native American: http://www.cyndislist.com/native.htm
Polish Genealogical Society of America: http://feefhs.org/pol/frg-pgsa.html
Quebec and Francophone: http://www.francogene.com/quebec/amerin.html
Romanian American Heritage Center: http://feefhs.org/ro/frg-rahc.html
Slovak World: http://feefhs.org/slovak/frg-sw.html
Slavs, South: Cultural Society: http://feefhs.org/frg-csss.html
Syrian and Lebanese Genealogy: http://www.genealogytoday.com/family/syrian/
Syria Genealogy: http://www.rootsweb.com/~syrwgw/
Tibetan Genealogy:
http://www.distantcousin.com/Links/Ethnic/China/Tibetan.html
Turkish Genealogy Discussion Group:
http://www.turkey.com/forums/forumdisplay.php3?forumid=18
Ukrainian Genealogical and Historical Society of Canada:
http://feefhs.org/ca/frgughsc.html
Unique Peoples: http://www.cyndislist.com/peoples.htm Note: The Unique
People's list includes: Black Dutch, Doukhobors, Gypsy, Romani, Romany &
Travellers, Melungeons, Metis, Miscellaneous, and Wends/Sorbs

Genealogy, (General):

Ancestry.com: http://www.ancestry.com/main.htm?lfl=m
Cyndi's List of Genealogy on the Internet: http://www.cyndislist.com/
Cyndi's List is a categorized & cross-referenced index to genealogical resources on the Internet with thousands of links.
DistantCousin.com (Uniting Cousins Worldwide)
http://distantcousin.com/Links/surname.html
Ellis Island Online: http://www.ellisisland.org/
Family History Library: http://www.familysearch.org/Eng/default.asp
http://www.familysearch.org/Eng/Search/frameset_search.asp
(The Church of Jesus Christ of Latter Day Saints) International Genealogical Index
Female Ancestors: http://www.cyndislist.com/female.htm
Genealogist's Index to the Web: http://www.genealogytoday.com/GIWWW/?
Genealogy Web http://www.genealogyweb.com/
Genealogy Authors and Speakers: http://feefhs.org/frg/frg-a&l.html
Genealogy Today: http://www.genealogytoday.com/
My Genealogy.com: http://www.genealogy.com/cgi-bin/my_main.cgi
Scriver, Dr. Charles: The Canadian Medical Hall of Fame http://www.virtualmuseum.ca/Exhibitions/Medicentre/en/scri_print.htm
Surname Sites: http://www.cyndislist.com/surn-gen.htm
National Genealogical Society: http://www.ngsgenealogy.org/index.htm
United States List of Local by State Genealogical Societies: http://www.daddezio.com/society/hill/index.html
United States Vital Records List:
http://www.daddezio.com/records/room/index.html or
http://www.cyndislist.com/usvital.htm

Appendix C

Bibliography 1

Medical Writing Bibliography, courtesy of American Medical Writers Association. See this information and more at the American Medical Writers Association's Web site at: http://www.amwa-dvc.org/toolkit/index.shtml#1a

Books

Style Guides
American Medical Association Manual of Style, 9th edition. Baltimore, MD et al.: Williams & Wilkins, 1998. Contact information: www.wwilkins.com, 800–638–0672.

Medical English Usage and Abusage. Edith Schwager (AMWA member), Phoenix, AZ, Oryx Press, 1991. Contact information: www.greenwood.com, 800–225–5800.

Mathematics into Type, Ellen Swanson, American Mathematical Society, Providence, RI: 1999. Contact information: www.ams.org.

The Elements of Style, fourth edition, William Strunk Jr. and E.B. White, Boston et al: Allyn and Bacon, 2000. Contact information: www.abacon.com.

Arthur Plotnik, *The Elements of Editing: A Modern Guide for Editors and Journalists*, New York, NY: Collier Books, 1982. Contact information: www.abacon.com.

Chicago Manual of Style, 14th edition. Chicago and London: University of Chicago Press, 1993. Contact information: www.press.uchicago.edu.

About Writing
William Zinsser, *On Writing Well*, sixth edition. New York, NY: Harper Perennial, 1998. Contact information: www.harpercollins.com.

Robert J. Bonk, PhD, *Medical Writing in Drug Development: A Practical Guide for Pharmaceutical Research*, Haworth Press, 1998. Contact information: www.haworthpressinc.com. Selected by Doody's Journal as one of the best health science books of the year!

Articles

"The Science of Science Writing," George D. Gopen and Judith A. Swan, *American Scientist*, Volume 78, November-December 1990.

"Clinical Trials: An Overview," Hardeo Sahai, Anwer Khurshid, and Muhammad I. Ageel, *Applied Clinical Trials*, December 1996.

Medical Dictionaries

Dorland's Illustrated Medical Dictionary, 28th edition. Philadelphia et al.: W.B. Saunders Company, 1994. Contact information: www.harcourthealth.com/WBS.

Stedman's Medical Dictionary, 26th edition. Baltimore, et al: Williams & Wilkins. Contact information: www.lww.com.

Freelance Resources (top)

Books

Robert W. Bly, *Secrets of a Freelance Writer: How to Make $85,000 a Year*, New York, NY: Henry Holt and Company, 1990. Contact information: www.henry-holt.com, 888–330–8477.

Marian Faux, Successful Freelancing: *The Complete Guide to Establishing and Running Any Kind of Freelance Business*, New York, NY: St. Martin's Press, 1982. Contact information: www.stmartins.com.

Alexander Kopelman. *National Writers Union Guide to Freelance Rates & Standard Practice*. New York, NY, 1995. Contact info: www.NWU.com, 212–254–0279; NWU@netcom.com.

Articles

"A Marketing Primer for Freelance Medical Writers," Lori De Milto, *AMWA Journal*, Vol. 14, No. 2, Spring 1999.

Bibliography 2: Pharmacogenetics

News articles:

*   Scientific, Ethical Questions Temper Pharmacogenetics
    Karen Young Kreeger
    The Scientist, 15[12]:32, June 11, 2001

*   Pharmacogenetics Initiative Galvanizes Public and Private Sectors
    Paul Smaglik
    Nature, Volume 410, March 15, 2001

Scientific Journal Articles:

1: Am J Hum Genet. 2002 Jan;70(1):157–69. Epub 2001 Nov 26. Comment in: Am J Hum Genet. 2002 Nov;71(5):1242–7. Bayesian haplotype inference for multiple linked single-nucleotide polymorphisms.

2. Mol Biol Evol. 1990 Mar;7(2):111–22. Inference of haplotypes from PCR-amplified samples of diploid populations. Clark AG. Department of Biology, Pennsylvania State University, University Park 16802.

Nature Biotechnology Pharmacogenomics Supplement, Volume 16, Number 10, October 1998, is a 21 page supplement provides an introduction, commentaries, feature articles and resources relevant to pharmacogenomics. See Web site at: http://www.nature.com/cgi-taf/dynapage. taf?file=/nbt/journal/v16/n2s/index.html. Also see: Nature Biotechnology Supplement Oct. 1998. See the Web site http://www.nature.com/ cgi-taf/dynapage.taf?file=/nbt/journal/v16/n2s/index.html.
One drug does not fit all. p 1
Andrew Marshall
doi:10.1038/5133
Why pharmacogenomics? Why now? pp 2–3
David Housman & Fred D. Ledley

doi:10.1038/5134
Pharmacogenetics and drug metabolism pp 4–5
Simon Ball & Neil Borman
doi:10.1038/5135
Laying the foundations for personalized medicines pp 6–8
Andrew Marshall
doi:10.1038/5138

Getting the right drug into the right patient pp 9–12
Andrew Marshall

Bibliography 3:

Nutritional Genomics:

Contact the American Society for Nutritional Sciences, or see the articles on the Web at Nutrition.org at: http://www.nutrition.org/. Note that HighWire Press(TM) assists in the publication of **The Journal of Nutrition Online** and **nutrition.org**.

Check out the articles listed below at *The Journal of Nutrition's* online site at: http://www.nutrition.org/. They are among several additional articles published in the September 2003 Volume 133 Number 9 issue of *The Journal of Nutrition.*

X. Zhang, X. Shu, Y. Gao, G. Yang, Q. Li, H. Li, F. Jin, and W. Zheng
    Soy Food Consumption Reduces the Risk of Coronary Heart Disease in Chinese Women

W. S. Wolfe, E. A. Frongillo, and P. Valois
    Understanding the Experience of Food Insecurity by Elders Suggests Ways to Improve Its Measurement

J. Hodgson, A. Devine, I. Puddey, S. Chan, L. Beilin, and R. Prince
    Tea Intake is Inversely Related to Blood Pressure in Older Women

A. K. Campbell, J. W. Miller, R. Green, M. N. Haan, and L. Allen
    Plasma Vitamin B-12 Concentrations in an Elderly Latino Population Are Predicted by Serum Gastrin Concentrations and Crystalline Vitamin B-12 Intake

A. T. Merchant, F. B. Hu, D. Spiegelman, W. C. Willett, E. B. Rimm, and A. Ascherio
> **Inverse Relationship between B Vitamin Supplements and Peripheral Arterial Disease Risk in Men**

B. Bartali, S. Salvini, A. Turrini, F. Lauretani, C. R. Russo, A. M. Corsi, S. Bandinelli, A. D'Amicis, D. Palli, J. M. Guralnik, and L. Ferrucci
> **The Association of Age and Disability with Dietary Intake**

B. T. Larson, D. F. Lawler, E. L. Spitznagel, and R. D. Kealy
> **Improved Glucose Tolerance with Lifetime Diet Restriction Favorably Affects Disease and Survival in Dogs**

E. S. Ford and A. H. Mokdad
> **Dietary Magnesium Intake among U.S. Adults: Findings from the National Health and Nutrition Examination Survey 1999–2000**

N. Pellegrini, M. Serafini, B. Colombi, D. Del Rio, S. Salvatore, M. Bianchi, and F. Brighenti
> **Total Antioxidant Capacity of Plant Foods, Beverages, and Oils Consumed in Italy Assessed by Three Different in Vitro Assays**

E. Naumann, J. Plat, and R. P. Mensink
> **Changes in Serum Concentrations of Non-Cholesterol Sterols and Lipoproteins in Healthy Subjects Do Not Depend on the Ratio of Plant Sterols to Stanols in the Diet**

J. G. Bell, D. R. Tocher, R. J. Henderson, J. R. Dick, and V. O. Crampton
> **Substitution of Marine Fish Oil with Linseed and Rapeseed Oils in Diets for Atlantic Salmon (Salmo Salar) affects Muscle Fatty Acid Composition: Restoration of Fatty Acid Composition Following 'Washout' with Fish Oil**

D. Ludwig
> **Glycemic Load Comes of Age**

Public education on nutrigenomics is available if you know where to look. If you're researching pet or farm animal diets, look at the company called Research Diets Incorporated. You can write to them at: 20 Jules Lane, New Brunswick, NJ 08901 U.S.A. See the site for **Research Diets at: http://www.researchdiets.com/**.

Human Genome

Adams, Julian, (editor), **Convergent Issues in Genetics and Demography**, (Oxford University Press, New York, 1990).

Brody, Tom, **Nutritional Biochemistry**, (Academic Press, San Diego, 2nd edition, 1999). There is a good discussion about "Nutrition methodology", including dot blots, molecular cloning, and DNA sequencing.

Brooks, William Keith, **The Law of Heredity: A Study of the Cause of Variation, and the Origin of Living Organisms**, (J. Murphy & Company, Baltimore, 1883).

Brown, Michael S., **Time Bombs in the Human Genome: Exploding Triplets That Cause Disease**, Medical Grand Rounds series, (University of Texas Southwestern Center, Dallas, 1993). This book is about the amplification of DNA trinucleotide repeats within the human genome. This can cause diseases such as Myotonic Dystrophy, Fragile X, and Muscular Atrophy.

Buckley, John J., **Genetics Now: Ethical Issues in Genetic Research**, (University Press of America, Washington, D.C., 1978).

Zallen, Doris Teichler, **Does It Run in the Family? A Consumer's Guide to DNA Testing for Genetic Disorders**, (Rutgers University Press, New Brunswick, New Jersey, 1997).

Zlinskas, Raymond A, and Balint, Peter J., (editors), **The Human Genome Project and Minority Communities: Ethical, Social, and Political Dilemmas**, (Praeger, Westport, Conneticut, 2000).

Classics in Molecular Genetics:

Watson, James D. **Molecular Biology of the Gene**, (W.A. Benjamin, Inc., New York, 1965, 2nd edition 1971, 3rd edition 1978, 4th edition 1987). This is the first edition of the "classic" textbook on molecular biology. At the time it was written, the genetic code was just being completely deciphered.

Watson, James D. **The Double Helix**, (W.A. Benjamin, Inc., New York, 1968, the "Norton Critical Edition" of this was published in 1980, edited by Gunther Stent, with reprints of some of the original papers.). This is a fun, very readable, "gossipy" account of the discovery of the DNA double helix. Of course, it is very biased, but nonetheless it makes good reading, and is very insightful into the personalities and politics involved in solving the basic structure of DNA.

Watson, J.D. and Tooze, J., **THE DNA STORY—A Documentary History of Gene Cloning** (W.H. Freeman and Company, San Francisco, 1981). This is kind of like a "scrapbook", with newspaper clippings, old letters, and lots of interesting stories about the beginning of genetic engineering.

The Human Genome in Europe: Scientific, Ethical, and Social Aspects, (Academie Royale de Medicine de Belgique, Bruxelles, 1995). This book is based on the proceedings of a conference in Brussels, Palais des academies, 18–19 September, 1995, by the Commission of the European Communities.

*   *   *

Bibliography : 4 General:
DNA Testing and Genetics.

A Biologist's Guide to Analysis of DNA Microarray Data Steen Knudsen/Hardcover/Wiley, John & Sons, Incorporated/April 2002

Advances and Opportunities in DNA Testing and Gene Probes Business Communications Company Incorporated (Editor)/Hardcover/Business Communications/September 1996

African Exodus, The Origins of Modern Humanity Stringer, Christopher and Robin McKie. Henry Holt And Company 1997

An A to Z of DNA Science: What Scientists Mean when They Talk about Genes and Genomes Jeffre L. Witherly, Galen P. Perry, Darryl L. Leja/Paperback/Cold Spring Harbor Laboratory Press/September 2002

An Introduction to Forensic DNA Analysis Norah Rudin, Keith Inman/Hardcover/CRC Press/December 2001

Archaeogenetics: DNA and the population prehistory of Europe, Ed. Colin Renfrew & Katie Boyle. McDonald Institute Monographs. Cambridge, UK, Distributed by Oxbow Books UK. In USA: The David Brown Book Company, Oakville, CT. 2000

Cartoon Guide to Genetics Gonick, Larry, With Mark Wheelis: Paperback/HarperInformation/July 1991

DNA Detectives, The—Working Against Time, novel, Hart, Anne. Mystery and Suspense Press, iuniverse.com paperback 248 pages at http://www.iuniverse.com or 1-877-823-9235.

DNA for Family Historians (ISBN 0-9539171-0-X). Savin, Alan of Maidenhead, England, is author of the 32-page book. See the Web site: http://www.savin.org/dna/dna-book.html

DNA Microarrays and Gene Expression Pierre Baldi, G. Wesley Hatfield, G. Wesley Hatfield/Hardcover/Cambridge University Press/August 2002

Microarrays for an Integrative Genomics Isaac S. Kohane, Alvin Kho, Atul J. Butte/Hardcover/MIT Press/August 2002

Does It Run in the Family?: A Consumers Guide to DNA Testing for Genetic Disorders Doris Teichler Zallen, Doris Teichler-Zallen, Doris Teichler Zallen/Hardcover/Rutgers University Press/May 1997

Double Helix, The: A Personal Account of the Discovery of the Structure of DNA James D. Watson/Paperback/Simon & Schuster Trade Paperbacks/June 2001

Genes, Peoples, and Languages Luigi Luca Cavalli-Sforza, Mark Seielstad (Translator).

Genetic Witness: Forensic Uses of DNA Tests DIANE Publishing Company (Editor)/Paperback/DIANE Publishing Company/April 1993

History and Geography of Human Genes, The [ABRIDGED] L. Luca Cavalli-Sforza, Paolo Menozzi (Contributor), Alberto Piazza (Contributor).

How to DNA Test Our Family Relationships Terry Carmichael, Alexander Ivanof Kuklin, Ed Grotjan/Paperback/Acen Press/November 2000

Introduction to Genetic Analysis Anthony J. Griffiths, Suzuki, Lewontin, Gelbart, David T. Suzuki, Richard C. Lewontin, Willi Gelbart, Miller, Jeffrey H. Miller/Hardcover/W. H. Freeman Company/February 2000

Jefferson's Children: The Story of One American Family Shannon Lanier, Jane Feldman, Lucian K. Truscott (Introduction)/Hardcover/Random House Books for Young Readers/September 2000

Medical Genetics Lynn B. B. Jorde, Michael J. Bamshad, Raymond L. White, Michael J. Bamshad, John C. Carey, John C. Carey, Raymond L. White, John C. Carey/Paperback/Mosby-Year Book, Inc./July 2000

Molecule Hunt, The: Archaeology and the Search for Ancient DNA Martin Jones/Hardcover/Arcade/April 2002

More Chemistry and Crime: From Marsh Arsenic Test to DNA Profile Richard Saferstein, Samuel M. Gerber (Editor)/Hardcover/American Chemical Society/August 1998

1996, Quest For Perfection—The Drive to Breed Better Human Beings, Maranto, Gina. Scribner, 1996

Our Molecular Future: How Nanotechnology, Robotics, Genetics, and Artificial Intelligence Will Transform Our World Mulhall, Douglas./Hardcover/ Prometheus Books/March 2002

Paternity—Disputed, Typing, PCR and DNA Tests: Index of New Information Dexter Z. Franklin/Hardcover/Abbe Pub Assn of Washington Dc/January 1998

Paternity in Primates: Tests and Theories R. D. Martin (Editor), A. F. Dickson (Editor), E. J. Wickings (Editor)/Hardcover/Karger, S Publishers/December 1991

Queen Victoria's Gene: Hemophilia and the Royal Family (Pbk) D. M. Potts, W. T. Potts/Paperback/Sutton Publishing, Limited/June 1999

Redesigning Humans: Our Inevitable Genetic Future Stock, Gregory./ Hardcover/Houghton Mifflin Company/April 2002

Rosalind Franklin: The Dark Lady of DNA, Brenda Maddox/Hardcover/ HarperCollins Publishers/October 2002

Schaum's Outline Of Genetics Susan Elrod, William D. Stansfield/Paperback/ McGraw-Hill Companies, The/December 2001

Seven Daughters of Eve, The: The Science That Reveals Our Genetic Ancestry. Sykes, Bryan. ISBN: 0393323145 Publisher: Norton, W. W. & Company, Inc. May 2002

Stedman's OB-GYN & Genetics Words Ellen Atwood (Editor), Stedmans/ Paperback/Lippincott Williams & Wilkins/December 2000

*   *   *

Bibliography 5 :
Genealogy.

A Bintel Brief: Sixty Years of Letters From the Lower East Side to the Jewish Daily Forward. Metzker, Isaac, ed Doubleday and Co. 1971. Garden City, NY

Climbing Your Family Tree: Online and Offline Genealogy for Kids IRA Wolfman,   Tim   Robinson   (Illustrator),   Alex   Haley (Introduction)/Paperback/Workman Publishing Company, Inc./October 2001

Complete Beginner's Guide to Genealogy, the Internet, and Your Genealogy Computer Program Karen Clifford/Paperback/Genealogical Publishing Company, Incorporated/February 2001

Complete Idiot's Guide(R) to Online Geneology Rhonda McClure/Paperback/ Pearson Education/January 2002

Creating Your Family Heritage Scrapbook : From Ancestors to Grandchildren, Your Complete Resource & Idea Book for Creating a Treasured Heirloom. Nerius, Maria Given, Bill Gardner ISBN: 0761530142 Published by Prima Publishing, Aug 2001

Cyndi's List: A Comprehensive List of 70,000 Genealogy Sites on the Internet (Vol. 1 & 2) Cyndi Howells/Paperback/Genealogical Publishing Company, Incorporated/June 2001.

Discovering Your Female Ancestors: Special strategies for uncovering your hard-to-find information about your female lineage. Carmack, Sharon DeBartolo. Conference Lecture on Audio Tape: Carmack, Sharon DeBartolo.

Folklife and Fieldwork: **A Layman's Introduction to Field Techniques.** Bartis, Peter. Washington, DC: Library of Congress, 1990.

Genealogy Online for Dummies Matthew L. Helm, April Leigh Helm, April Leigh Helm, Matthew L. Helm/Paperback/Wiley, John & Sons, Incorporated/February 2001

Genealogy Online Elizabeth Powell Crowe/Paperback/McGraw-Hill Companies, November 2001

History From Below: How to Uncover and Tell the Story of Your Community, Association, or Union. Brecher, Jeremy. New Haven: Advocate Press/Commonwork Pamphlets, 1988.

My Family Tree Workbook: Genealogy for Beginners Rosemary A. Chorzempa/Paperback/Dover Publications, Incorporated/

National Genealogical Society Quarterly 79, no. 3 (September 19991): 183–93

"**Numbering Your Genealogy: Sound and Simple Systems**." Curran, Joan Ferris.

Oral History and the Law. Neuenschwander, John. Pamphlet Series #1. Albuquerque: Oral History Association, 1993.

Oral History for the Local Historical Society. Baum, Willa K. Nashville: American Association for State and Local History, 1987.

Scrapbook Storytelling: **Save Family Stories & Memories with Photos, Journaling & Your Own Creativity** Slan, Joanna Campbell, Published by EFG, Incorporated, ISBN: 0963022288 May 1999

"**The Silent Woman: Bringing a Name to Life**." NE-59. Boston, MA: New England Historic Genealogical Society Sesquicentennial Conference, 1995.

The Source: A Guidebook of American Genealogy Alice Eichholz, Loretto Dennis Szucs (Editor), Sandra Hargreaves Luebking (Editor), Sandra Hargreaves Luebking (Editor)/Hardcover/MyFamily.com, Incorporated/February 1997

To Our Children's Children: Journal of Family Members, Bob Greene, D. G. Fulford 240pp. ISBN: 038549064X Publisher: Doubleday & Company, Incorporated: October 1998.

Transcribing and Editing Oral History. Nashville: American Association for State and Local History, 1991.

Using Oral History in Community History Projects. Buckendorf, Madeline, and Laurie Mercier. Pamphlet Series #4. Albuqueque: Oral History Association, 1992.

Unpuzzling Your Past: The Best-Selling Basic Guide to Genealogy (Expanded, Updated and Revised) Emily Anne Croom, Emily Croom/Paperback/F & W Publications, Incorporated/August 2001

Writing a Woman's Life. Heilbrun, Carolyn G. New York: W.W. Norton, 1988

Your Guide to the Family History Library: How to Access the World's Largest Genealogy Resource Paula Stuart Warren, James W. Warren/Paperback/F & W Publications, Incorporated/August 2001

Your Story: A Guided Interview Through Your Personal and Family History, 2nd ed., 64pp.ISBN: 0966604105 Publisher: Stack Resources, LLC

*   *   *

Bibliography 6:

List of Published Paperback Books in Print Written by Anne Hart
Also See:
http://www.newswriting.net or email: newswriting@hotmail.com
Alternate site: http://annehart.tripod.com/booklist.html
Reviews: http://annehart.tripod.com
Audio and Video: http://www.newswriting.net/writingvideos.htm

1. Predictive Medicine for Rookies: Consumer Watchdogs, Reviews, & Genetics Testing Firms Online   ISBN: 0-595-35146-8

2. Popular Health & Medical Writing for Magazines: How to Turn Current Research & Trends into Salable Feature Articles ISBN: 0-595-35178-6

3. Title: Writing 45-Minute One-Act Plays, Skits, Monologues, & Animation Scripts for Drama Workshops: Adapting Current Events, Social Issues, Life Stories, News & Histories

ISBN: 0-595-34597-2

4. Cutting Expenses and Getting More for Less: 41+ Ways to Earn an Income from Opportune Living

ISBN: 0-595-34772-X

5. Title: How to Interpret Family History and Ancestry DNA Test Results for Beginners: The Geography and History of Your Relatives

ISBN: 0-595-31684-0

6. Title: Cover Letters, Follow-Ups, and Book Proposals: Samples with Templates

ISBN: 0-595-31663-8

7. Title: Writer's Guide to Book Proposals: Templates, Query Letters, & Free Media Publicity

ISBN: 0-595-31673-5

8. <u>Search Your Middle Eastern and European Genealogy:</u> In the Former Ottoman Empire's Records and Online

ISBN: 0-595-31811-8

9. <u>Ancient and Medieval Teenage Diaries:</u> Writing, Righting, and Riding for Righteousness

ISBN: 0-595-32009-0

10. Is Radical Liberalism or Extreme Conservatism a Character Disorder, Mental Disease, or Publicity Campaign?—A Novel of Intrigue—

ISBN: 0-595-31751-0

11. How to Write Plays, Monologues, and Skits from Life Stories, Social Issues, and Current Events—for all Ages.

ISBN: 0-595-31866-5

12. Title: How to Make Money Organizing Information

ISBN: 0-595-23695-2

13. Title: How To Stop Elderly Abuse: A Prevention Guidebook
ISBN: 0-595-23550-6

14. Title: How to Make Money Teaching Online With Your Camcorder and PC: 25 Practical and Creative How-To Start-Ups To Teach Online
ISBN: 0-595-22123-8

15. Title: A Private Eye Called Mama Africa: What's an Egyptian Jewish Female Psycho-Sleuth Doing Fighting Hate Crimes in California?
ISBN: 0-595-18940-7

16. Title: The Freelance Writer's E-Publishing Guidebook: 25+ E-Publishing Home-based Online Writing Businesses to Start for Freelancers
ISBN: 0-595-18952-0

17. Title: The Courage to Be Jewish and the Wife of an Arab Sheik: What's a Jewish Girl from Brooklyn Doing Living as a Bedouin?
ISBN: 0-595-18790-0

18. Title: The Year My Whole Country Turned Jewish: A Time-Travel Adventure Novel in Medieval Khazaria
ISBN: 0-75967-251-2

19. Winning Resumes for Computer Personnel, Barron's Educational Series, Inc. ISBN: 0-7641-0130-7

20. Title: The Day My Whole Country Turned Jewish: The Silk Road Kids
ISBN: 0-7596-6380-7

21. Title: Four Astronauts and a Kitten: A Mother and Daughter Astronaut Team, the Teen Twin Sons, and Patches, the Kitten: The Intergalactic Friendship Club
ISBN: 0-595-19202-5

22. Title: The Writer's Bible: Digital and Print Media: Skills, Promotion, and Marketing for Novelists, Playwrights, and Script Writers. Writing Entertainment Content for the New and Print Media.
ISBN: 0-595-19305-6

23. Title: New Afghanistan's TV Anchorwoman: A novel of mystery set in the New Afghanistan
ISBN: 0-595-21557-2

24. Title: Tools for Mystery Writers: Writing Suspense Using Hidden Personality Traits

ISBN: 0-595-21747-8

25. Title: The Khazars Will Rise Again!: Mystery Tales of the Khazars

ISBN: 0-595-21830-X

26. Title: Murder in the Women's Studies Department: A Professor Sleuth Novel of Mystery

ISBN: 0-595-21859-8

27. Title: Make Money With Your Camcorder and PC: 25+ Businesses: Make Money With Your Camcorder and Your Personal Computer by Linking Them.

ISBN: 0-595-21864-4

28. Title: Writing What People Buy: 101+ Projects That Get Results

ISBN: 0-595-21936-5

29. Title: Anne Joan Levine, Private Eye: Internal adventure through first-person mystery writer's diary novels

ISBN: 0-595-21860-1

30. Title: Verbal Intercourse: A Darkly Humorous Novel of Interpersonal Couples and Family Communication

ISBN: 0-595-21946-2

31. Title: The Date Who Unleashed Hell: If You Love Me, Why Do You Humiliate Me?

"The Date" Mystery Fiction

ISBN: 0-595-21982-9

32. Title: Cleopatra's Daughter: Global Intercourse

ISBN: 0-595-22021-5

33. Title: Cyber Snoop Nation: The Adventures Of Littanie Webster, Sixteen-Year-Old Genius Private Eye On Internet Radio

ISBN: 0-595-22033-9

34. Title: Counseling Anarchists: We All Marry Our Mirrors—Someone Who Reflects How We Feel About Ourselves. Folding Inside Ourselves: A Novel of Mystery

ISBN: 0-595-22054-1

35. Title: Sacramento Latina: When the One Universal We Have In Common Divides Us

ISBN: 0-595-22061-4

36. Title: Astronauts and Their Cats: At night, the space station is cat-shadow dark

ISBN: 0-595-22330-3

37. Title: How Two Yellow Labs Saved the Space Program: When Smart Dogs Shape Shift in Space

ISBN: 0-595-23181-0

38. Title: The DNA Detectives: Working Against Time

ISBN: 0-595-25339-3

39. Title: How to Interpret Your DNA Test Results For Family History & Ancestry: Scientists Speak Out on Genealogy Joining Genetics

ISBN: 0-595-26334-8

40. Title: Roman Justice: SPQR: Too Roman To Handle

ISBN: 0-595-27282-7

41. Title: How to Make Money Selling Facts: to Non-Traditional Markets

ISBN: 0-595-27842-6

42. Title: Tracing Your Jewish DNA For Family History & Ancestry: Merging a Mosaic of Communities

ISBN: 0-595-28127-3

43. Title: The Beginner's Guide to Interpreting Ethnic DNA Origins for Family History: How Ashkenazi, Sephardi, Mizrahi & Europeans Are Related to Everyone Else

ISBN: 0-595-28306-3

44. Title: Nutritional Genomics—A Consumer's Guide to How Your Genes and Ancestry Respond to Food: Tailoring What You Eat to Your DNA

ISBN: 0-595-29067-1

45. Title: How to Safely Tailor Your Food, Medicines, & Cosmetics to Your Genes: A Consumer's Guide to Genetic Testing Kits from Ancestry to Nourishment

ISBN: 0-595-29403-0

46. Title: One Day Some Schlemiel Will Marry Me, Pay the Bills, and Hug Me.: Parents & Children Kvetch on Arab & Jewish Intermarriage

ISBN: 0-595-29826-5

47. Title: Find Your Personal Adam And Eve: Make DNA-Driven Genealogy Time Capsules

ISBN: 0-595-30633-0

48. Title: Creative Genealogy Projects: Writing Salable Life Stories

ISBN: 0-595-31305-1

49. Title: Power Dating Games: What's Important to Know About the Person You'll Marry

ISBN: 0-595-19186-X

50. Dramatizing 17th Century Family History of Deacon Stephen Hart & Other Early New England Settlers: How to Write Historical Plays, Skits, Biographies, Novels, Stories, or Monologues from Genealogy Records, Social Issues, & Current Events for All Ages

ISBN: 0-595-34345-7

51. Creative Genealogy Projects: Writing Salable Life Stories

ISBN: 0-595-31305-1

52. Problem-Solving and Cat Tales for the Holidays: Historical—Time-Travel—Adventure

ISBN: 0-595-32692-7

53. 801 Action Verbs for Communicators: Position Yourself First with Action Verbs for Journalists, Speakers, Educators, Students, Resume-Writers, Editors & Travelers

ISBN: 0-595-31911-4

54. Writing 7-Minute Inspirational Life Experience Vignettes: Create and Link 1,500-Word True Stories

ISBN: 0-595-32237-9

55. Large Print Crossword Puzzles for Memory Enhancement: Neuron-Growing Stimulation for the Age-Wise Brain

ISBN: 0-595-35663-X

56. Middle Eastern Honor Killings in the USA: (A Thriller)

ISBN: 0-595-36066-1

57. Tracing Your Baltic, Scandinavian, Eastern European, & Middle Eastern Ancestry Online: Finnish, Swedish, Norwegian, Danish, Icelandic, Estonian, Latvian, Polish, Lithuanian, Greek, Macedonian, Bulgarian, Armenian, Hungarian, Eastern European & Middle Eastern Genealogy (All Faiths)

ISBN: 0-595-35773-3

58. Middle Eastern Honor Killings in the USA (A Thriller)

ISBN: 0-595-36066-1

59. Infant Gender Selection & Personalized Medicine: Consumer's Guide

ISBN: 0-595-36539-6

60. Writing, Financing, & Producing Documentaries: Creating Salable Reality Video: ISBN: 0-595-36633-3

61. How to Turn Poems, Lyrics, & Folkloreinto Salable Children's Books: Using Humoror Proverbs: ISBN: 0-595-36735-6

Appendix D

Where to Find Speech Transcripts

Consumers can dialogue with the food industry. Brainstorm how you can work together to research and communicate about the "shift in thinking about the way food is processed, packaged, and marketed in the U.S," according to an online report in the Harvard Public Health NOW, published biweekly. Meetings and a July 2003 conference drew the food industry, public health professionals, scientists, nutrition researchers, and anyone else present. FDA has critical issues to handle—such as safety and security of food and edible imports—in addition to helping consumers improve nutrition. That's why FDA added more than 650 new food safety monitors in the field.

In a speech before Harvard School of Public Health, Remarks by Mark B McClellan, MD, PhD, Commissioner, Food and Drug Administration presented on July 1, 2003 included, "We need your input on how we can use these new means to achieve the greatest improvements in public health protection, with the least possible disruption and added costs for the foods we regulate. And we must do it quickly, because these new measures have to be implemented before the end of the year."

Consumers—your help is needed. Here's how to find out more information. Research speech archives and obtain a transcript of the Speech before Harvard School of Public Health, Remarks by Mark B McClellan, MD, PhD, Commissioner, Food and Drug Administration presented on July 1, 2003. For more information about news or conferences, see: Harvard Public Health NOW, published biweekly by the Office of Communications, Harvard School of Public Health, 665 Huntington Ave., SPH 1–1312A, Boston, Massachusetts 02115. Or click on the Web site at: http://www.hsph.harvard.edu/now/jul11/conference.html Search the archives of the Harvard School of Public Health at: http://www.hsph.harvard.edu/now/archives.html.

Contact the Office of Communications, Harvard School of Public Health if you are writing on public health issues for the media. Since numbers could change, click on the Web site at: http://www.hsph.harvard.edu/communications.html to find current names of people to contact, phone, fax, or email addresses that will help you get the expert information you need to write your article.

Contact Information

Director of Communications
Kresge 1015
677 Huntington Avenue
Boston, MA 02115

Media inquiries

Assistant Director of Communications
Kresge 1014
677 Huntington Avenue
Boston, MA 02115

General Mailing Address:

Harvard School of Public Health
Office of Communications
677 Huntington Avenue
Boston, MA 02115

Appendix E

Permissions:

——Original Message——
From: "Andrew Y. Silverman, M.D., Ph.D."
To: "Anne Hart"
Sent: Thursday, June 30, 2005 1:14 PM
Subject: Gender Selection Chapter

Dear Anne,

You have my permission to publish the chapter as written. I understand that I will not receive financial compensation for the chapter from sales of the book, but I also understand that I retain the copyright of my own material.

Sincerely,

Andrew Y. Silverman, M.D., Ph.D.

Dear Anne,

You have permission to use the primer text and the photo of the DNA molecule for your book on DNA testing for genealogists. Please prominently credit the U.S. Department of Energy Human Genome Program as the source for both and also include our website for more information on the Human Genome Project and its applications: www.ornl.gov/hgmis. Yes, you can use the *Dictionary of Genetic Terms* at the end of the online version of the Primer. Please provide source citations when you use each part of the document. We would appreciate having a copy of your book when it is completed.

Sincerely,
Denise Casey

Denise K. Casey
Science Writer/Editor
Human Genome News
Human Genome Management Information System
Oak Ridge National Laboratory
1060 Commerce Park, MS 6480
Oak Ridge, TN 37830
865/574–0597; Fax: 865/574–9888; Email: caseydk@ornl.gov
HGMIS World Wide Web URL: http://www.ornl.gov/hgmis
Sponsor: U.S. Department of Energy

Harry Ostrer, M.D.
Professor of Pediatrics, Pathology, and Medicine
Director, Human Genetics Program
New York University School of Medicine
550 First Avenue, MSB 136
New York, NY 10016
tel 212 263–7596
fax 212 263–3477

——Original Message——
From: Frederic Abramson
To: Anne Hart
Sent: Wednesday, July 23, 2003 2:21 PM
Subject: Re: Permissions

Hi Anne

I would be honored to have the article included, and the quote about the viruses.

Fredric

           *   *   *

——Original Message——
From: Peter Sprague
To: Anne Hart
Sent: Wednesday, August 20, 2003 12:21 PM
Subject: Re: query

Ms. Hart,

Permission granted as long as we are cited as the source.

Regards,

PFS

Peter Frost Sprague
Editorial Director
Physician's Weekly LLC
490 Highway 33 West
Englishtown, NJ 07726
732–792–1558 Office
732–792–1568 or 732–786–1165 Fax

Index

978-0-595-36539-5
0-595-36539-6